PRAISE FOR KICKASS

"There is so much information out there on the internet about keto. From what I have seen, 75% of it is incorrect, confusing and not based in science. This book will help you drown out all the noise and get the facts you need to get started."

– Jessyca Reynolds, Ketofied and half my size

I'm loving this. You make Keto easy to understand and follow.

– Danette Hess

If you're looking for an amazing and easy plan, this is the book for you!
There are weekly meal plans with recipes and shopping lists (these shopping lists are awesome! Not only do you see what you need to buy each week, there are notes that tell you which item goes in which recipe!), information about exercising along with ideas to get you started, and so much more!
Trust me, you NEED this!

– Kimberly Hull

Ketovangelist LLC

2358 Williamson Road

Lockhart, TX 78644

www.ketovangelist.com

www.kickassketo.org

Layout and Design by Rekka Jay.

ISBN-10: 0-9998262-0-4
ISBN-13: 978-0-9998262-0-1

Digital books are available from kickassketo.org

KICKASS KETO

YOUR 28-DAY QUICK START GUIDE TO

HEALTH, FAT-BURNING, & WEIGHT LOSS

BRIAN WILLIAMSON, CARRIE BROWN, AND REKKA JAY

CONTENTS

The food you eat can be either the safest and most powerful
form of medicine or the slowest form of poison.
- Dr. Ann Wigmore

Let food be your medicine, and medicine be your food.
- Hippocrates

You are what you eat.
- Anonymous

This book is dedicated to **you**,
because you're **awesome!**

PART 1: YOUR KETO SOLUTION

It's no secret: what you eat has tremendous impact on your health and well-being. But the world is awakening to the terrible truth of what we've been told about healthy eating over the past 60 years. The dogmatic insistence that fat is bad and carbs are harmless has begun to erode.

Thanks to the tireless and often unsung efforts of a small band of researchers and scientists, the tide is turning. The keto revolution has started, and if you're reading this, you're part of the rebellion.

It's not enough for researchers and scientists to discover (or rediscover) the healthiest foods and lifestyles. Change like this requires you. It requires you to enjoy the lifestyle, the food, and the improvements to your physical, mental, and emotional health. And it takes you sharing all those things with the people around you.

That's how we will win this fight. Because we are tired of watching people slowly poison themselves with the terrible food that the orthodox establishment insists is healthy. It isn't. And if you care about your health, you're going to want to read this book closely. You're going to want to implement the plans. (You're also going to realize that Carrie makes keto delicious.)

So read on, fellow rebel. Challenge yourself to get healthy. And don't worry, this book will make it easy and fun.

WHY KETO?

Obesity and overweight have been on the rise for decades, but over the past six decades, the trend has increased significantly. Several recent reports indicate as many as two out of every three Americans are overweight or obese, and there doesn't seem to be a slow down in sight. Of course, it's no coincidence that this increase has coincided with the nutritional dogma that fat is bad, grains are good, and all you need to do to lose weight is exercise more and eat less.

Of course, all three of those things are wrong. And we'll be discussing the factors which brought us to this particular state of unhealthy living a little later, but suffice it to say strong personalities, bad science, and governmental bureaucrats are the real reason we've been given bad nutritional guidance for the past 60 years. People have been eating that way for over two generations and people have been getting fatter. It's not enough to "eat clean." You have to eat the right things.

Luckily, not everyone was suckered by the bad science. A small remnant of researchers and scientists continued to demonstrate that dietary fat is not only not the cause, but is part of the solution for overall health. That's where the ketogenic diet comes in. The ketogenic diet is a high-fat, moderate-protein, and very low-carb way of eating. Just like that, believe it or not, you can lose body fat, gain energy, improve health, and feel incredible.

PROBLEMS WITH THE STANDARD AMERICAN DIET

In the world of nutrition, there are two things that provide nutrients to your body. **Micronutrients** are vitamins and minerals. **Macronutrients**, or macros, are bigger molecules which are used for energy. There are three kinds of macros: fat, protein, and carbohydrate. **The Standard American Diet (SAD) is <u>very</u> high in carbs and <u>very</u> low in fat.** And that might not seem like a problem, but it really is. Ignoring, for the moment, the fact obesity and overweight have skyrocketed over the course of the past 60 years –the same amount of time the low-fat, high-carb SAD way of eating has been pushed by experts and governments – a diet consisting of very high carbs and very low fats has been linked to diabetes, cardiovascular disease, heart disease, stroke, Alzheimer's, epilepsy, autoimmune disorders, systemic inflammation, cancer, gastrointestinal disorders, and many other illnesses, disorders, and diseases.

Many of those disorders are directly tied to obesity and overweight.

But it gets worse. The vast majority of the carbs (up to 65%) in the SAD are manufactured, processed, or refined. For fear of fats, recipes are flooded with sugar to increase their palatability.

Hoping to eat like that and still lose body fat is like trying put out a house fire with a hose that sprays gasoline.

The primary connection between the incredibly high number of carbs and the incredibly high rate of obesity and overweight (and all the associated illnesses) can be summed up with one primary factor: Insulin levels.

High levels of carbohydrates in your diet will result in high levels of insulin in your blood. And high levels of insulin, when experienced over time, will lead directly to obesity, sickness, and worse.

Insulin is a hormone produced by the pancreas. Its primary job is energy partitioning. Without insulin, your cells would not receive any energy. Body cells require insulin in order to use blood glucose. But when insulin levels are very high, and they stay very high, your cells become resistant to insulin. So it takes more and more insulin to feed your cells the same amount of energy. More insulin means more problems, because insulin also stores your unused energy, as fat molecules, into fat cells.

So, to put it simply, if you increase the amount of insulin you have in your blood, you will increase the amount of fat you store. If you decrease the amount of insulin in your blood, you will decrease the amount of fat you store.

The ketogenic diet is the best way to lower insulin levels, stay satisfied, and get healthy.

BURN FAT, NOT SUGAR

If high levels of carbs are bad, because they trigger high levels of insulin, then where are you supposed to get your energy? Isn't sugar the way we get energy in our bodies?

Well, yes and no. Sugar is a simple form of energy, but it's not the only form of energy. It's not even the best, or preferred, form of energy in your body. For that, we turn to fat. Your body is designed to burn stable fats. That's why it converts excess energy to saturated fat for storage in your cells! So here's where the ketogenic diet comes in.

When your body starts to burn fat for fuel, it creates special molecules known as **ketones**. When your body has a certain level of ketones built up in the blood, you're in a state known as nutritional ketosis. This state is the basis of the ketogenic diet. Having enough ketones in your body to supply your energy needs means you don't have to worry about eating any sort of carbohydrate (which will be converted to sugar, spike your insulin, and make you gain fat). Since you are minimizing your carbohydrate intake, with a ketogenic diet, you are allowing your body to minimize the amount of fat that it stores. Not only that, but the lowered levels of insulin also help alleviate the long list of illnesses you read about earlier.

We hear stories, every day, through our numerous Facebook groups and through our websites, of people who have lost 50 pounds, 70 pounds, 100 pounds, or more, just by switching to a well-formulated ketogenic diet.

The carbs are a killer and fat is where it's at.

To get into a state of nutritional ketosis, a few things have to happen. First, you have to reduce your dietary carbohydrate intake. Second, you figure out your protein requirement. Third, use that protein requirement to give you an idea of how much fat you should eat every day.

Don't worry, we'll help you determine those targets, but suffice it to say that getting into a state of ketosis isn't terribly difficult.

With the exception of fiber, your body will convert all the carbs you eat to sugar (glucose). When there's sugar present in your blood, your body will burn that sugar for energy. Any unused sugar will be stored as fat.

But when you cut the availability of glucose to near-zero, your body begins to burn fat for fuel. Without carbs in your diet, you force your body to choose a different fuel source, and since fat is the most abundant fuel source in your body, your liver starts to metabolize fat molecules and make them into ketones. If you've got extra weight in the form of fat cells, your body begins to treat that as a fuel tank.

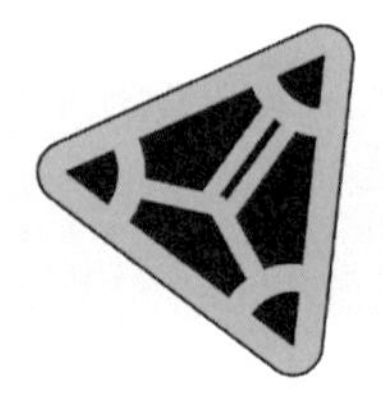

To delve deeper into the theory behind keto, check out our huge library of articles, available free at www.ketovangelist.com

KETOGENIC DIET PRINCIPLES

The ketogenic diet (keto) has been around for many years in various forms for therapeutic purposes. However, we won't be addressing those formulations in this book, because the primary focus of this book is weight loss and weight management. So when we talk about keto, we are referring to a specific formulation of macros.

As you read previously, carbs, protein, and fats are all known as macros, which is short for macronutrients. They are the building blocks for your body and your body's energy.

Keto is low in carbs, moderate or adequate in protein, and high in fat.

Keto also eliminates starches and sugars (both natural and processed).

Beware the Fad Followers

If you've already tried to follow a keto diet by using information gathered from across the internet, you probably don't need us to tell you there's a **lot** of contradictory information out there.

We suspect there are a few reasons for this:

1) People are quick to write advice articles, build blogs, write cookbooks, and offer coaching for an audience without fully understanding a ketogenic diet for themselves.

2) People mistake other low carb diets for "as good as" keto. Atkins, Paleo, Low Carb, South Beach; the terms aren't interchangeable, and neither are the ingredients. These search terms often get lumped together in an effort to catch the searches of as many audiences as possible.

3) Bad information spreads faster than good. Probably it's because some of that bad information is what people want to hear (IIFYM, CKD, to name a couple concepts we do **not** recommend).

We **wish** we could scrub the web of misleading and confusing information, but that's not possible (or legal). The only thing we can do is try to educate our Ketovangelists to a higher level of understanding and, as a result, performance.

Even if you think you know keto, we strongly recommend you begin the Kickass Keto 28-Day Quick Start challenge by forgetting everything you've read online, and prepare to refill that empty cup with sound science and simple strategies for success during the 28 days of this challenge, and beyond.

Low Carb

Low carb has lots of different meanings for lots of different people. And it makes sense that it would, especially considering the fact that the average person consumes 75% to 80% of their food in the form of carbs. If you eat 2000 calories per day, that would equate to something like 1500 to 1600 calories in the form of some kind of carb. That's roughly 375 to 400 grams of carbs per day. So when you hear about something being "low carb," it's possible to be in the 150 to 200 grams per day range, and be lower in carbs than the average person. But keto keeps carbs even lower than that.

General advice is to **keep your carb intake around 20 grams per day or less**, especially in the beginning. As you progress, and you become more of a keto veteran, you'll be able to increase your carb intake if you want, but we don't recommend anyone going above 50 grams per day.

So when we talk about keto being low-carb, we're talking VERY low, because the carbs are mucking up your hormones.

What are "Net" Carbs?

Net carbs can be a source of controversy, but the theory behind measuring **net carbs** instead of **total carbs** is based on your body's digestive process. Insoluble fibers (the type folks recommend to resolve or ward off constipation) don't get digested by your body.

When folks switched to extremely low carb diets, they worried their avocados and other veggies would take up too much of their carb allowance for the day. Not wanting to discourage folks from eating their greens, the concept of net carbs was born.

Total Carbs (g) – Insoluble Fiber (g) = Net Carbs (g)

The sticky wicket, when it comes to net carbs, is manufacturers have begun to produce packaged "low carb" foods which rely on very high amounts of Insoluble Fibers (not always from quality sources) in order to call themselves "low carb." This deceptive labeling has led some folks to gastric or insulinemic trouble.

In our Facebook groups, some people track total carbs, and others track net carbs. There's a third option: track net carbs for whole foods, and total carbs from packaged products. How you track is up to you, and what works best for your body.

Moderate Protein

For some reason, a lot of people seem to think protein is a tricky thing. We don't. There are a couple of reasons for that, but mostly it's because things shouldn't be too complicated. If there's an opportunity to simplify things, you should take it. Luckily, when it comes to protein, we'll do it for you. Keep in mind all macro guidelines are just that, **guidelines**. They are suggestions and starting points.

The real answer to your macros will be uncovered through some trial and error as you move toward your goal.

As a guideline, your protein intake should be as follows:

Females: 50 to 75 grams per day

Males: 100 to 120 grams per day

Everyone is different. Lots of people find tremendous success by eating less protein than the minimum number we listed. Some people can eat more than the max and still make progress. It's not a one-size-fits-all. You have to take an active roll in figuring out what works for you, but this is a great place for you to start.

A Closer Look at a "Healthy" Whole Foods Diet

The nutrition world has a lot of competing ideas about what it means to be healthy. One of the most prevalent is the concept of eating "Whole Foods," which isn't necessarily a bad thing. However, it's very important to understand, just because a food is "whole" doesn't make it healthy. The best example would be whole grains. We are inundated by advertising that depicts whole grains as the pinnacle of healthy food choices. The problem with grains is they result in high levels of insulin. And high levels of insulin result in people getting fat and sick.

Just because a food item is taken from the ground does not make it healthy for you to eat. That's a romantic notion, but it's far from the truth. That's not to say all vegetables are bad, either. There are plenty of vegetables which fit perfectly within a ketogenic diet. Just don't be fooled into thinking grains and starches do.

High Fat

Thanks to the scientific community, we have guidelines for macros and formulations, making the high-fat portion of keto easy. The general idea for nutritional ketosis, which is what you want to achieve for weight loss and weigh management, is to **keep your daily fat intake within a range of 65 to 80 percent of your food**.

Wait: But Isn't Fat Bad For You?

That's a bit of a trick question, actually. Not all fat is created equal, and some fats are better than others. Vegetable oils, which are hydrogenated and unstable, and not great for you. However, all animal fats (butter, ghee, beef, pork, etc.) are great. These kinds of fats are classified as **saturated fats**. Saturated fat has been demonized for many years, but is only dangerous when consumed with high levels of carbohydrates. Saturated fats are stable fats, which are fantastic and you shouldn't be afraid of them. Another great source for saturated fat is coconut oil, which we highly recommend. A couple other great sources of fats are avocado oil, olive oil, and macadamia nuts. These are classified as mono-unsaturated fats, and they are also fantastic. Mixing different kinds of fats together, like butter and olive oil, for example, creates a wonderful combination. Not only does it taste great, but it contains a great mix of good fats.

The common thought of fats as unhealthy couldn't be further from the truth. If you are consuming saturated and mono-unsaturated fats, you really cannot go wrong. The idea that fats are bad for you is based upon faulty science, misinterpretation, and politics.

Look at it this way: if using fat as your primary fuel source was unhealthy, then every single person who, like us, has lost body fat would be getting unhealthier as we got skinnier. When you lose weight, you are living on the energy of that body fat. When you lose 50 pounds of body fat, you are burning 50 pounds of saturated fat. We don't hear anyone complaining! In fact, medical professionals all recommend it. So, ultimately, the whole idea of fat being unhealthy is just plain illogical.

Luckily, it's easy to figure out how much fat that actually is. And it's related to your protein intake. If you eat 50 grams per day of protein, your fat intake should fall within a range of 50 to 100 grams per day. If you eat 80 grams per day of protein, your fat intake should fall within a range of 80 to 160 grams per day. If you eat 120 grams of protein per day, your fat intake should fall within a range of 120 to 240 grams per day.

Did you notice anything about the fat numbers we recommend? If you noticed **the fat recommendation is between a 1:1 and 2:1 ratio of your protein**, then you get a high five. That's exactly what it should be to fulfill that requirement of 65 to 80 percent of daily energy. It's really that simple.

So let's recap:

Carbs:	**20 grams or less per day**
Protein:	**50 to 75 grams (females) or 100 to 120 grams (males) per day**
Fat:	**Between 1:1 and 2:1 to your protein grams**

BENEFITS OF KETO

Lose weight

We become fat mostly because of hormones, not calories, and eliminating carbs and increasing fats will work wonders to stabilize hormone levels. Many people who choose keto eat the same amount of food they always have and still lose body fat. An added bonus is with keto, it's much easier to lose belly fat. The adage is true that abs are made in the kitchen...

The Ketovangelist Kitchen.

Mental clarity and focus

In addition to allowing you to lose body fat, stabilizing other regulatory hormones allows your brain to burn ketones instead of sugar. Ketones are a much cleaner fuel, so there is far less "rust" or "byproducts" in your brain. You will experience mental clarity and the lifting of the "brain fog" many people don't even recognize, because they've been walking around in it for so long.

So you'll not only look better, you'll think better, too.

Emotional stability

You'll also be happier. At least that's what most people report. Because your brain isn't stressed by a bad fuel source, and your hormones are regulated with an efficiency unlike what a SAD lifestyle allows, keto definitely allows you to feel better.

Appetite control

One of the scariest things for new keto people is to discover they are no longer slaves to sugar. Sugar burns fast, and your body will want more and more, because it's addictive. In turn, your appetite hormones go wild, and you're hungry all the time. Keto has the opposite effect. As it balances your appetite hormones, primarily leptin and ghrelin, your appetite drops. It startles people, because they have been stuck in a vicious cycle of blood sugar spikes and drops for so long, they don't know what it's like to not be hungry. But it's incredibly freeing when you switch to keto, because you will actually be in control of your health.

Disease treatment

As we listed earlier, keto has a long track record of successfully treating diabetes, cardiovascular disease, heart disease, stroke, Alzheimer's, epilepsy, autoimmune disorders, cancer, gastrointestinal disorders, and many other illnesses, disorders, and diseases.

Decreased inflammation

If there was one thing which seems to be present in every case of illness, it's systemic inflammation. Inflammation happens when your immune system causes swelling to parts of your body, because it thinks it's under acute "attack." When inflammation is present for long periods of time, your health declines rapidly.

Ketones have a natural resistance to the primary enzyme responsible for inflammation.

The types of foods in a well-formed ketogenic diet are also less inflammatory than common ingredients on a SAD menu.

So choosing keto means you'll be even healthier on the inside.

Increased energy

We guarantee you'll experience increased energy once you've been keto for a while and transition completely into a fat-burning state. Your body will start operating like it was designed to and you'll be untethered from constant hunger for sugar. Plus you'll be eating plenty of awesome food, so you should be energized to get up and move. It's not unusual, at all, for keto folks to become athletes, even those who never even considered it before.

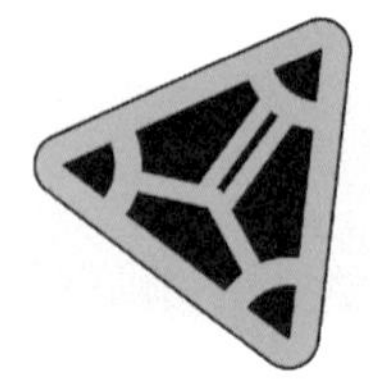

Witness impressive success stories by joining the Ketogenic Success Facebook Group at facebook.com/groups/ketogenicsuccess

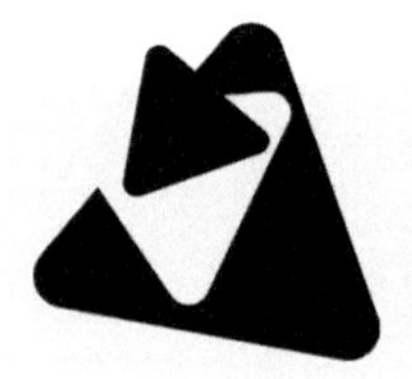

You can join the amazing community at ketovangelistunlimited.com to interact with like-minded people having enormous success with keto, further fine-tuning their lives for ultimate health and performance.

PART 2: PILLARS OF HEALTH

So that brings us to the main thrust of this book. Our challenge to you...our Kickass Keto challenge.

Simply put, we want you to use the recipes, food guide, nutrition guidelines, and information within this book to give a well-formed ketogenic diet a whole-hearted, disciplined try for at least 28 days, to see how easy it will be for you to lose weight (for some of you, it'll be probably be the first time anything has ever worked for your weight loss), get healthy, and feel great.

You've seen those ridiculous commercials touting how you can eat whatever you want and still lose weight, right? They always talk about how easy and simple it is.

And it never works.

And you probably blame yourself for it not working.

Well, this ain't that.

BEYOND THE "DIET" MENTALITY

Our expectations are that you will take the information we give you and put it to good, solid, disciplined work. **Because this isn't a miracle cure. It's a lifestyle change. It's a journey.**

And every journey, great and small, requires a first step. If you want to get to your destination, all you have to do is keep taking those steps, every day, until you get there.

And we are here to help you every step along the way. Whether you are a keto newbie, or you are a keto veteran, you will find something in this book to help you get on the right path and stay on the right path.

Whether your goals are big or small, whether you want to lose a lot of weight or a little, the detailed information in this book will help you get there. Because it got us where we wanted to go, and we've watched it help countless thousands of others who tell us, almost every day, about how they've used keto to lose weight and get healthy.

If you follow our advice, you will get results. It's that simple.

This book isn't just a list of meals to eat. It's detailed information about the fundamental pillars to a healthy lifestyle:

1. **Nutrition**
2. **Exercise**
3. **Sleep & Hydration**
4. **Mindset**
5. **Community**

Each of these pillars will be referenced, explained, and detailed in the chapters to come. And if you heed those chapters, you will see the results you want.

PILLAR 1: KETO NUTRITION

Because of the prevalence of the low-fat myth, and because of the mistaken "calories is how you get fat" myth, a lot of nutrition plans offer some of the most boring, bland food imaginable.

The problem with this is two-fold. First, in order to make a lot of this kind of food palatable, they have to doctor it up, typically with sugar (if you remove the fat from food, it tastes awful, which leaves sugar as the only way to keep it tasty). Second, it makes it very easy for you to crave more unhealthy food. Whether it's because you aren't meeting your energy needs, or because you just don't like eating boring food, you are statistically more likely to stray from typical low-fat fare.

Keto meals are rich in healthy fats, which means you don't have to skimp on flavor in the slightest. Still, these old nutrition myths and problems linger with us from our previous attempts at weight loss and the dogma that most of us have been exposed to since grade school.

Nutrition is confusing. It doesn't have to be. It isn't supposed to be. But it is.

And that's because almost everything you've been taught about proper nutrition is wrong. The advice to avoid fats, get lots and lots of "healthy" grains, and sugar is okay "in moderation," is responsible for 90% of weight gain, health problems, not to mention frustration. You try a diet based upon these recommendations, and it doesn't work. Then this advice is repeated over and over, and you feel as if you're the problem. That it's all your fault. But it's not.

To make matters more confusing, the way to get back to health, and the way to start losing weight, is by going against the nutritional orthodoxy by making fat the primary component of your diet.

We've seen the frustration, and we understand. Our goal is to alleviate that frustration, and make it simple and easy for you to understand what keto is and how to implement it effectively as a lifestyle.

ALL ABOUT RATIOS

There are a lot of "sacred cows" in nutrition (no pun intended), none more so than the calorie hypothesis. Ask any ordinary nutritionist, dietary consultant, doctor, or medical researcher how people get fat and you will likely hear the same answer: People get fat because they take in more calories than they burn.

That's it. No discussion. No question. No problem.

That, in a nutshell, is the calorie hypothesis.

Except it's wrong. And it is dangerous.

If you ask any of these same folks how excess calories results in fat accumulation, you'll get less consistent and less confident answers. Some of them will throw out terms like "thermodynamics" or some other such ideas. Some will, flat out, not be able to explain how it happens (they are the honest ones), but they will all stick to their original answer: the calorie hypothesis.

The reason they are not really able to explain how excess calories adds to body fat is because there is no biological mechanism available to explain how calories cause weight gain. There is no molecule, no hormone, no enzyme, nothing biological available in the human body that takes "excess" calories and stores them as fat. It just doesn't happen. That's because a calorie isn't a physical thing. It's a form of measurement, in the same way that a kilogram or a mile is not a physical thing. They are all just measurements. If someone asked you to hand them "a pound," your answer would be, "a pound of what?"

A calorie is a measure of heat, more specifically, a measure of the amount of heat it takes one gram of water to increase by one degree celsius. When conventional wisdom tells you to eat 2000 calories, what does that even mean?

Focusing on an abstract measurement isn't going to make things easy for you. Focusing on food, however, will. When it comes to eating, "2000 calories of *what*?" is an excellent question. And keto gives you the answer. When you maintain a keto-friendly ratio of fat-to-protein-to-carb, you will be armed to have more success in your weight loss.

As we talked about in the previous chapter, fat, protein, and carbs are macronutrients, or macros. Each one of these macros produces a certain amount of heat when your body digests it. So when someone talks about the calories in fat, protein, or carbs, that is what they are referring to.

Carbohydrates have roughly 4 calories per gram. Protein, also, has about 4 calories per gram. Fat has somewhere in the neighborhood of 9 calories per gram. Incidentally, alcohol has about 7 calories per gram, but that's just a nice bit of trivia.

So one of the reasons that people fear fat is because it is calorically dense food. And if they believe calories are the way you get fat, then they want to remove that calorically dense item from your menu.

There is one final point of consideration in this, though. Inevitably, when we talk about calories, someone will insist that calories matter, and they always will. And there is truth in that, but it's not what most people think. The types of calories matter far more than the amount of calories. Different kinds of calories cause different hormonal responses in your body, insulin being the primary hormone which determines putting on body fat. So, by eliminating (or drastically reducing) the amount of certain calories (carbs), you are able to keep your hormones in check and reduce the likelihood of putting on body fat.

Not only that, but the truth is, there is no real, accurate way to measure your caloric intake and expenditure, so focusing on calorie quantity is really an exercise in futility.

The kinds of calories you eat matter far more than the amount. Because you can control the kinds of calories you eat. Setting your macros up in a ketogenic ratio is going to maximize your weight loss effectiveness.

Macros for Weight Loss

One of the great things (among many, many great things) about keto is that it's very flexible. You tailor things to what works best for you. You don't have to rearrange everything in your life to fit into some rigid "diet."

That flexibility starts with the macros. Since the primary focus for this book is on nutritional ketosis (as opposed to therapeutic ketosis), the macro breakdown for your food is going to be flexible.

We really want you to understand macros, so we're going to provide some details and examples below. Now...we will be talking about calories, but only as a reference point, and not as an actual nutritional consideration. Please don't be confused by that.

Okay, so let's figure out some macros for a hypothetical keto newbie. We'll call the newbie Chris. We'll start with protein (a very good place to start).

If Chris is female, she should start off her protein in the range of 50 to 75 grams per day. She will then add fat between a 1:1 and 2:1 ratio. So she'll be eating between 50 to 150 grams per day of fat. And she'll keep her carbs to 20 grams or below.

If Chris is male, he should start off his protein in the range of 100 to 120 grams per day. He will then add fat between a 1:1 and 2:1 ratio. So he'll be eating between 100 to 240 grams per day of fat. And he'll keep his carbs to 20 grams or below.

It's not more complicated than that. Flexible doesn't mean complicated. Some people will lose weight faster if they are on the higher range of dietary fat, and some people will lose weight faster if they are on the lower range of dietary fat. We recommend starting at the higher range and moving to the lower range as needed. Your protein intake will determine your fat intake. So it's best to start with a protein amount inside the respective range above, and that will lead to your fat amount.

No matter what, though, you're going to want to keep your carbs to 20 grams per day or less. One thing to keep in mind, too, regarding carbs, is you can use total carbs or net carbs in your measurements. Total carbs is simple: Add the carbs and that's that. Net carbs is a little more involved: Add the carbs and subtract fiber and non-caloric sweeteners (erythritol, stevia, or xylitol). Whichever method you choose (and plenty of people find success using either method), just keep it consistent.

Because keto is flexible, the recipes in this book stay within that flexible range. Every recipe is safely within the acceptable keto range of macros. Like we said, we have made it as easy as possible for you.

Keto Quotient

Rather than use Macros, which are often times difficult to determine due to improper labeling and other factors, Ketovangelist has a system of Certified Ketogenic labels to identify the quality of recipes and packaged food in terms of Ketogenic nutrition.

Keto Friendly (KF) Keto Approved (KA) Certified Ketogenic (CK)

For the best results during your Kickass Keto challenge, all of the recipes in this book are Certified Ketogenic.

Read more about Certified Ketogenic and the metrics of each rating at www.certifiedketogenic.com

Micronutrients

A quick word about micronutrients and keto. Most people know micronutrients as vitamins and minerals. They are important, obviously. But with the removal of the nutritional "noise" (i.e. carbs), your body will be far more efficient with how it uses vitamins and minerals. A well-rounded keto menu will have a complete micronutrient profile. **To put it simply, the only real micronutrients you may need to supplement are Vitamin C, Magnesium, and, to a lesser extent, Potassium.**

If you think you need more Vitamin C, you can put some lemon or lime juice in your water. If you think you need more Magnesium, you can order some Chelated Magnesium Glycinate from Amazon (we recommend between 400 to 800 mg per day). If you think you need more Potassium, you can cook vegetables in your meat drippings.

WHAT TO EAT

Now that you understand macros and how they should be portioned, the question becomes: What foods should you actually eat?

Healthy Fats

Examples of healthy fats are saturated and mono-unsaturated fats. Any fats from animals like beef, pork, dark meat poultry, dairy, fatty fish, or eggs are excellent. Coconut oil and red palm oil are also great sources of saturated fat. Olive oil and avocado oil are some of the best sources of mono-unsaturated fats. Macadamia, almond, and walnut oils are also great. Salmon is a fantastic source of great omega-3 fatty acid.

Protein

Quality protein can be found in beef, pork, poultry, eggs, fish, lamb, venison, and eggs. **The best kinds of proteins are "complete proteins," which contain all amino acids which cannot be created by your body.** Luckily, animal protein is a great source of complete protein.

Keto-Friendly Alternatives

This chart that provides Keto-friendly alternatives to high-carb favorite foods.

To train yourself not to look for familiar indulgences, this list is not a like-for-like substitution list.

This list also requires little to no cooking. There are many Ketofied versions of favorite high-carb snacks, so if you are willing to cook, there are tons of things out there you can have instead of the high-carb, SAD diet comfort foods.

TRADE:	FOR:
Potato Chips	Pork Rinds
Cookies	Dill Pickles
Lattes w Syrup	Coffee w HWC
Toast	Bread Cheese
Crackers	Cheese Crisps
Fruit	Berries or Sliced Avocado
Granola	Nuts

Vegetarians and vegans, please take note: While it is possible to get protein from some plant sources, we must re-emphasize they will not be complete proteins. Incomplete proteins (mostly from vegetables) are a combination of amino acids missing at least one of the essential amino acids. If you are a vegetarian or vegan, you may find it difficult to get adequate protein without the use of a protein powder supplement. However, no supplement will work as well as animal protein.

Keto-Friendly Vegetables

Vegetables come in a wide assortment of varieties, shapes, and sizes. **And, for the most part, you cannot go wrong with green, leafy vegetables.**

Other great keto options for vegetables are broccoli, cauliflower, celery, cucumbers, garlic, mushrooms, onions, tomatoes, zucchini, and most varieties of squash. Keep in mind, though, this isn't a complete list, and there are other keto-friendly vegetables available to you, but put simply, if the vegetable isn't high in carbs, it should be okay. Almost any fermented or pickled (not sweet) vegetable is great.

Keto-Friendly Fruits

Most fruits are far too high in natural sugar content to be keto-approved, but some varieties of berries are okay in small amounts. Blackberries, raspberries, strawberries, and cranberries, to name a few. Also, lemons and limes are perfectly okay.

Nuts and Seeds

Because most nuts are great sources of fat, many of them work as part of a keto diet. **The problem with nuts is they also contain carbs, and it's easy to over snack on them, so you need to be conscious of what you're eating and how much.** Macadamia nuts, almonds, brazil nuts, walnuts, pili nuts, and pecans are fine for the vast majority of people. It's probably a good idea to avoid cashews and pistachios. We would advise staying away from most seeds and seed oils.

Alcohol – That "Other Macronutrient"

Alcohol is a macronutrient with seven calories per gram. It's a byproduct of fermentation. The more distilled, and the fewer added ingredients, the less likely the alcohol will knock you out of ketosis.

An important thing to remember is to stay hydrated. Alcohol prevents that and leads to dehydration. That's what a hangover is, mostly, a lack of proper hydration. Our bodies become more efficient with water, so we need to keep water in good supply. If you choose to drink, make sure to consume two water drinks for every alcohol drink.

There's one final consideration for alcohol. It is, essentially, a poison. There is ample evidence to show how long-term use can damage the liver, kidneys, pancreas, and brain. Your body recognizes alcohol as something which must be metabolized immediately, and so long as alcohol is in your system, you will cease burning fat (nutritional or stored).

You may still register ketones after consuming alcohol, but as you can imagine, drinking is not something which will help you achieve your keto goals.

People with addictive personalities really should abstain from alcohol, period.

To get you started on your keto journey with the best chance for success, we do not include alcohol in the Kickass Keto plan.

A DAY OF KETO MEALS

A lot of nutrition and weight loss books include very rigid schedules and strict guidelines. Keto isn't like that. As we've mentioned, keto is fundamentally about freedom.

Generally speaking, we recommend eating larger meals, less often. This helps reduce blood sugar spikes, and therefore reduces the levels of insulin in your blood. And, as we've discussed, insulin is the main method for you to gain body fat. One thing a lot of life-long dieters find difficult about keto is there are very few hard and fast rules. We've discussed the macro breakdowns, and this book provides a full meal plan and a relatively complete list of keto foods. So, once you have those things down and know what foods work for you, there aren't a lot of other rules.

Most people experience a dramatic loss of appetite when they become keto. This is normal. You will experience the freedom of not craving food every couple of hours. Intermittent Fasting (IF) is also "baked in" with keto. That means you could possibly go 8, 10, 12, or more hours without eating, because you do not have an appetite and you feel great. There is no reason to force-feed yourself, since you will begin to listen to your body and eat only when you're hungry.

So a day of keto meals could look something like this:

First meal: Coffee with fat (butter, coconut oil, and/or MCT oil)

Second meal (if necessary): A handful (approximately an ounce) of macadamia nuts

Third meal (if necessary): Creamy Cajun Sausage Skillet

It's that simple. Of course, if you feel the urge to snack, you can choose something small but satiating from the Meal 2 Selections list on page 124. If you feel the urge to continuously snack, you are not eating enough during your meals.

On page 66 you'll find a list of keto-friendly whole foods. You might find it helpful, while you're still getting the hang of this lifestyle, to print the list out and keep it with you.

How Much and When

As we've stressed in other sections, everyone is different and it is extremely difficult to create a meal plan to work for everyone right out of the box. Your appetite, food sensitivities, ingredient preferences, schedule, and budget are things we simply cannot predict.

Our menus allow for up to three meals per day. We have been trained by nutritional dogma to look for a snack or small meal every couple of hours, but the act of eating triggers insulin release, and eating more than three times per day minimizes the dramatic benefits of keeping insulin low.

Don't be surprised to find yourself less and less hungry over the course of the Kickass Keto challenge. If you do not need to eat three meals each day, skipping one is entirely acceptable. We designed our menus to accommodate bigger appetites, to keep you from having to make extra trips to the store which might lead to temptation (especially when shopping hungry).

The shopping lists for each week indicate which recipes ingredients are called for, to better help you adjust if you find, after the second week, you are consistently not eating all three meals.

If you incorporate workouts into your day, we recommend eating **after** your workout. This may not sound logical based on everything you've been told about exercise and fueling your body, but trust us and give it a shot. You can always bring along a baggy of pre-portioned nuts in case you're not ready for a fasted workout just yet.

BECOMING FAT-ADAPTED

When your blood has a large enough supply of sugar, your body will deal with that sugar first. It'll burn what it can for energy and insulin will help store the rest as fat. But when you decrease the amount of blood sugar to the point where your body no longer has enough to supply its energy needs, your body will send signals to your liver to start metabolizing fat and using ketones for fuel. When your liver produces a certain amount of ketones, you are considered "in ketosis."

Your liver will receive molecules known as triglycerides, and split them apart. Each triglyceride contains three fat molecules which share a "backbone" made up of another kind of molecule called glycerol. Your liver will convert these newly freed fat molecules to ketones, so your body and brain can use them for fuel. Because your brain has specific barriers, fat cannot be used as a direct fuel source. Your brain can only burn ketones or sugar. It cannot burn fat, because fat molecules are too big to cross the blood-brain barrier. So your liver starts to produce lots of ketones when there is not enough sugar in your blood, and these ketones are used to fuel most of your brain and your muscles.

So when people talk about being in ketosis, they are referring to the ketones in their body which are available for fuel. The phrase "kicked out of ketosis" means the opposite: some factor (usually eating too many carbs) has caused the ketone reading to drop below the measurement required for ketosis.

However, being in ketosis is not the same thing as being fat-adapted (aka keto-adapted). They are related, but they are different. You become fat-adapted when your body's muscles begin using fat, and not ketones, as their primary fuel source.

It takes a certain period of time for your body to get used to burning fat for fuel and, in that time, your muscles and your brain will compete for ketones.

If you are in ketosis for a period of time (and that period of time is different for everyone), your muscles will begin to learn how to burn fat (not just ketones) for fuel. At that point, the competition between your muscles and your brain stops, and you are fat-adapted.

The transition period, though, between decreasing dietary carbs and your muscles being able to burn fat for fuel can be difficult, and has a name: The Keto Flu. A lot of people feel sluggish, run down, unfocused, and tired during this time. Headaches or body aches are not uncommon. Of course, not everyone experiences it to the same degree, and some don't show any sort of symptoms at all.

If you are experiencing the keto flu, the main things to remember are:

1. Get enough sodium – At least 2 teaspoons per day of good salt, such as Himalayan or Celtic Gray. Table salt has been stripped of nutrients, so try to get the good stuff.

2. Get enough water – Stay hydrated.

3. Get enough rest – 6 ½ to 8 hours per night is important.

4. Trust the process - It's worth it.

REPLACE YOUR ELECTROLYTES

When you eliminate carbs, your body will "flush" a lot of water, and when it flushes a lot of water, a lot of your electrolytes go with it. It's important to keep those replenished to minimize any bad symptoms. You can also keep keto-friendly foods around which are higher in sodium, magnesium, and potassium:

Dill Pickles + the brine (pickle juice)

Sauerkraut Watercress Cheese Spinach

Mushrooms Avocado Greek Yogurt (full-fat, plain)

Many don't have an appetite during the keto flu, and prefer to add salt and lemon juice to a glass of water, or drink pickle juice.

TESTING YOUR KETONES

There are three kinds of ketones in your body, and each one has a specific method of measurement. These are beta hydroxybutyrate (BHB), acetoacetate (AcAc), and acetone. Thy are measured, respectively, via blood, urine, and breath. So you'd use a blood meter to measure BHB, urine strips to measure AcAc, and a breath meter to measure acetone.

Each one of the methods of measuring has pros and cons.

Urine test strips are cheap and easy to find at most drug or grocery stores. However, urine strips are the least reliable method of testing your ketone levels, and for several reasons. First, a strip measures AcAc, which your body will likely stop eliminating through urine as you stay in ketosis and your body becomes more efficient at using ketones. Second, it measures ketone volume relative to liquid in your urine, so if you're dehydrated, the urine strips will show higher levels of ketones, but only because you're dehydrated. It isn't an accurate way to measure your ketone levels. Just because the stick is dark doesn't mean you're in ketosis.

Blood testing is very accurate, but it's also more expensive. Since testing your blood requires a blood meter, you need to get one which tests glucose **and** ketones, because not all do. You also need to maintain a supply of ketone blood test strips, and they can range from $3 - $7 per strip (though the price has started to come down and will hopefully continue to do so). So if you wanted to test your ketone levels 5 times per day, it could cost you as much as $15 - $35 per day. That's $450 - $1050 per month. Ouch! Oh, and speaking of ouch, you have poke your finger to draw blood every time you want to test – not a pleasant experience.

Breath testing is accurate and one device can be used repeatedly by multiple people for a long time. The only drawback to breath meters, is the initial price, which can be somewhere between $165 - $200 for the Ketonix, while the Levl starts at $600. But you can use it multiple times per day and it's accurate each time, so you can definitely get your money's worth out of them.

	Urine Strips	Blood Meter	Breath Analyzer
Pros	Cheap Convenient Painless	Accuracy	Reliable Reusable Computer/App tracking
Cons	Very low accuracy	Expensive Painful	Large Initial Investment
Measures	AcAc (wasted ketones)	BhB (available ketones) Blood Glucose (needs BG strips)	Acetone (used ketones)

Having said all that, though, we really want you to understand you don't need to measure your ketones in order to lose weight. In fact, plenty of people never measure anything and reach their goals. If you find you do better by testing, or if you have a medical reason to want a consistently high ketone level, then test.

If you don't need to test, and you're making progress toward your goals, don't test and trust that it's working.

PILLAR 2: EXERCISE

Exercise is an important part of any weight loss journey. In this chapter, we'll review best practices for exercise and provide recommendations for your 28-day program and beyond.

In recent decades, because of the faulty calorie hypothesis, exercise was used as tool for weight loss, often the primary tool.

"Eat less and move more." Sound familiar?

But in keto, we know the primary factor responsible for fat accumulation is increased levels of insulin and insulin resistance. If that can be corrected, more fat can be mobilized from cells and used as fuel.

Insulin sensitivity increases with heavy resistance training (less-so with steady-state cardio), but only if you give your cells a break from high levels of insulin (hyperinsulinemia).

Along with insulin, cortisol, leptin, and ghrelin (to name just a few) are also affected by exercise and exercise intensity. Cortisol is present when the intensity increases. Leptin levels will drop with exercise. Ghrelin levels will increase with exercise.

More to the point, the hormonal adjustments are temporary and will return to your "normal" levels post-workout...and you'll probably be hungry because of it. So it's not the exercise which causes fat loss, it's the diet.

That doesn't mean exercise cannot be fueled by body fat. In fact, if you're in ketosis, almost all your exercise **will** be fueled by your body fat, but calories aren't the key factor.

So if calories are not the mechanism for fat gain or loss, then what role, if any, does exercise play in achieving health and fitness goals? Several, but they may not be the ones you expect.

But before we get into that, we just need to bring up a question that everyone needs to answer for themselves:

WHY DO YOU WANT TO EXERCISE?

What goal will exercising help you achieve? If you don't know the answer, you're almost guaranteed to fail in your exercise life. A ketogenic lifestyle incorporates a unified approach to all aspects in order to achieve something better.

So, having said that, and having asked you to consider why you would choose to torture yourself, let's talk about exercise.

Exercise fosters many positive impacts as part of a healthy, ketogenic lifestyle.

STRESS RELIEF

Let's start with the first: stress relief. This is the most important reason for regular exercise.

Exercise triggers a lot of biochemical responses, such as increasing cortisol, the hormone responsible for dealing with stress, and increasing norepinephrine, a neurohormone associated with mood and other things.

These increases cause us to relax, because when they drop back down to normal levels, the stress, for lack of a better phrase, melts away.

The longer, and more frequently, you exercise, the less hormone is needed and the lower your resting stress rate. Regular exercise allows for widespread, systemic stress relief.

This, of course, is empirically provable. People just feel better after exercise.

There is an upper limit, though, to your stress threshold. If you engage in vigorous aerobic activities for extended periods of time, for many days in a row, you will begin to actually **increase** your stress. So don't over do it.

MENTAL ACUITY

The second role for exercise is mental acuity. The same neurohormone which aids in stress relief, norepinephrine, is responsible for increased memory and focus. The large amount of norepinephrine which release into your system during exercise goes to work making you smarter. Even if you think you're too busy to add exercise into your routine, taking the time to physically work your body will bring improvements to your professional life, and you'll be able to do more and feel less mental fatigue doing it.

When you add exercise to a keto diet, which already improves your mental functions (because your brain **really** loves running on ketones), you become unstoppable.

FUN

The third and, we think, most common reason for exercise is fun. Now, we will say not everyone agrees with which exercise or the degree to which it is fun, but people tend to stick to an exercise regimen when they enjoy something about it.

If it was complete and total torture, with no demonstrable benefits, people would not exercise at all. You need to figure out what kinds of exercise you enjoy enough to keep them up.

Everyone is different. As with any lifestyle change, there is no one-size-fits-all situation. Some people like to run, walk, bike, swim, lift weights, do Crossfit, or jiu-jitsu. Some like to do different combinations of any of the above or others (kayaking, rowing, rock climbing, hiking, etc.).

The **kind** of exercise isn't important. **Exercising** is. If you are in a routine that you don't enjoy, which you don't find fun, then you need to try something else. Brian would play basketball every day, or do jiu-jitsu, or run, but the idea of biking makes him want to eat his own face. He couldn't stand it if he had to kayak or row every day. But that's just Brian, and that's okay. He found something he liked and stuck with it.

Brian's wife loves to play tennis, and also runs several days per week.

So what do you like? Don't know? That's okay. Just try some different things out and see how you like them. Wanna run? Get some good shoes and try it. If you don't like it (assuming you try with real effort), at least you have yourself some new shoes. If you don't like to run, try something else. Some people love the elliptical machine or stair climber. If that appeals to you, try it.

You get the idea. No matter what you decide to do, get out there and move. Your brain will thank you for it.

Once you find something you like, we have one final recommendation. There are three forms of exercise which work very well with the keto lifestyle: HIIT, LIA, and LHS. We'll talk more about each in the next sections.

Get Started Now: Simple, Go-To Exercise Circuits. No Gym Required.

Planks	Contract your abs to help you hold your back flat and bear your weight on your forearms, elbows, and toes (or knees, to start).
Split Squat	Hold your shoulders square and step into a lunge with your feet in one line. Keep your knees behind your toes as you dip with the front leg. Experiment with your arm position to work on your balance.
Push-Ups	Contract your abs to help you hold your back flat while lowering your chest toward the floor and pressing with your arms to raise back to the starting position. Experiment with your hand and arm positions to work different muscles in your arms.
Ab Vacuums	While standing, sitting, or on hands and knees, contract your abdomen muscles as you exhale. Imagine you are pulling your navel toward your spine. Hold your breath or breathe mindfully (inflating your chest instead of your stomach) while you hold your abs tight. If you do breathe, re-tighten the contraction with each exhalation.

HIIT (HIGH INTENSITY INTERVAL TRAINING)

High Intensity Interval Training is perhaps the single best exercise you can do for fat loss, stress relief, and feeling great. HIIT is quick, hard, and rewarding. When you hear "high intensity", that's exactly what you should expect. Engaging in HIIT is not for the timid, and there's a great possibility you will hate every minute of it. Until it's over. Then you'll be glad you did it.

HIIT is some powerful stuff and a little goes a long way. With HIIT, you don't spend a lot of time during your workout (5 minutes or less, 10 minutes if you have a warm up), but you will feel as accomplished as if you completed a triathlon.

What's an interval?

Interval training is when you go all-out for a short spurt, and then rest, and then do it again. The most common is the **Tabata Protocol**, which lasts 4 minutes, but don't let the short time fool you. You go all-out for 20 seconds, rest for 10 seconds, and repeat that sequence for 8 rounds. You can do this with body exercises, sprints, biking, or any other of a long list of things. It provides a very intense, very good workout which doesn't require hours of precious time.

The beneficial effects are pronounced:

- Intervals boosts growth hormone.
- Intervals improve muscle efficiency (so you burn more fat).
- Intervals reduce the levels of blood triglycerides after a meal.
- Intervals improve your insulin sensitivity.

For free resources on exercise, check out The Ketogenic Athlete

Website: theketogenicathlete.com

Facebook Group: facebook.com/groups/theketogenicathlete

Podcast: theketogenicathlete.com/category/podcast

As we said earlier, if you aren't ready to try sprinting, you can do body weight exercises. For example, to really work you out, try eight 20-second intervals of any of the following exercises, alternated with ten seconds of rest.

Jump Lunges

Push-Ups

Squats

Burpees

Plank To Push-Up

Spiderman Push-Up

Mountain Climbers

Bicycle Crunch

Russian Twist

Side-To-Side Push-Up

Squat Kicks

Firecrackers

Speed Skaters

Inch Worms (Stationary)

Pick four of these and perform the intervals twice for a total of eight. It's that simple. Try this and we guarantee you will feel it. HIIT training really is incredible.

LIA (LOW-INTENSITY AEROBICS)

Low-intensity aerobic exercise is the second part of the three necessary pieces of keto fitness.

This one is very simple to explain: Walk.

For an hour or so, two to three times per week, if you can. If not, as much as you're able (and try to find time for the hour walks). And that's it.

You get all the benefits of the aerobic exercises (like running, biking, swimming, etc.) without the struggle to maintain a certain pace, and running the risk of injury. Your heart and lungs get a workout, but without the intensity and stress. It seems too easy, but walking is a fantastic way to help lower blood pressure, lower blood triglycerides, decrease stress, increase mental focus, improve aerobic capacity, and a host of other things.

But mostly, it's a great way to think about things you want to think about. All day long, most of us have to think about things other people want us to think about, whether they are our kids or our bosses or our spouses or friends. That's not necessarily a bad thing, but it is nice to have some time where you can just concentrate on things you want to think about.

If you like walking with a friend, it's a great time to catch up on the events of the day and bond.

If you incorporate this into your schedule, you'll see results (or at least feel them) quickly. And you'll wonder why didn't do it sooner.

LHS (LIFTING HEAVY STUFF)

Lifting heavy stuff is the single best form of exercise for any person interested in improving their health. For years, we were told, and believed, it was impossible to gain muscle and lose fat at the same time. The reason for this thinking was a belief in the incorrect calorie hypothesis. If the calorie hypothesis was true, the only way to gain muscle would be to have a calorie surplus, and the only way to lose fat would be to have a calorie deficit. Since math is...math, it is a logical impossibility to be in a state of both surplus and deficit at the same time.

But the underlying paradigm is incorrect; we enlarge our muscles by stressing and resting them, and we lose fat by correcting our nutrition. So it is very possible to lose fat and gain muscle at the same time. All it takes is a little bit of discipline, some heavy stuff, and a pig-headed devotion to the ketogenic lifestyle.

The only way that we put on muscle is to increase the stress on our muscles to the point where they must grow in order to accommodate the stress. Excess calories don't do that. Lifting very heavy things does that. When you stress your muscles, you break them, and the body builds them back up bigger, so they can handle the stress. It is important, however, to have enough dietary protein to heal the injured muscle cells. So if you are attempting to gain muscle, you will need to check your protein levels to make sure you getting enough to build the muscle.

(Here's a hint: Chances are, your protein levels are plenty high).

At the same time, while building muscle, if you are eating a well-formulated keto diet, you will burn through your body fat. But you'll also recover quicker, feel less sore, and increase strength faster.

So what should you do to build muscle? Well, the answer to that question has filled shelves and shelves of books (and an entire podcast; here's a shameless plug for The Ketogenic Athlete). But we'll simplify it: Heavy, compound movements.

That simply means using the heaviest weights you can move, and using movements that stress large areas of muscles. So what are some example of compound exercises?

Here's a list:

Bench Press (Chest, Triceps, Lats)

Squat (Quads, hamstrings, Glutes)

Pull-Ups (Lats, Biceps)

Military Press (Delts, Triceps, Traps)

Push-Ups (Chest, Triceps, Lats)

Deadlift (Quads, Hamstrings, Forearms, Lower Back, Lats)

If you concentrate on those compound movements, and lift as heavy as you can, you will put on muscle and gain strength.

It's important to note by lifting "heavy," we don't mean go straight for power lifting records. Heavy is a term relative to your capacity, and it will change as you improve.

So there you go. It is absolutely possible to gain muscle while losing fat. It just takes a combination of disciplined exercise of lifting heavy weights and eating a ketogenic diet.

EXERCISE MYTHS

The worldwide fitness industry generates more than $78 billion each year, and there's no sign it's going to slow down any time soon. There's a lot of money at stake, and not every company in the industry is interested in the truth. Many of them will say anything to get you to buy from them. Whether it's the latest "must-have" supplement (which is likely full of fillers and other questionable ingredients), the newest machine which will end up as a clothes hanger, or the newly discovered secret nutrition plan (which is the same exact nutrition plan they were selling last year, in a different color), there are a lot of myths and mistakes being passed off as truth. So we've listed some of the biggest offenders below, along with our take.

Fat Loss Is About Calories

This one has a lot of different variations, but it boils down to the same idea. The basic logic is this: you lose fat by consuming less calories than you expend. So to lose fat, all you have to do is eat less and exercise more. This has been the standard advice for the past 60 years, the same 60 years which have seen massive increases in obesity and metabolic disease.

The reason it doesn't hold true is because there are two ways to kick-start your body's **starvation** response: restricting your calories and increasing your energy expenditure. So by taking the advice of the "experts" who say calorie restriction is how you lose fat, you're actually telling your body that you're starving. Your body will respond in one of two ways: eat everything in sight or to depress your metabolism.

By restricting calories and increasing your energy output, you are signaling your body to hold on to the resources it has stored because (in primal terms) you have been hunting and hunting, and were unable to successfully find food.

The truth is the **fat loss** we work so hard to achieve is 80%-90% about nutrition and **not** about exercise. And it's got nothing to do with the number of calories you eat.

You Can Spot Reduce (Or, Sit-Ups Give You Abs)

This is a particular pet peeve of ours, because it is so demonstrably false. The idea behind this myth is you can work out a particular muscle group in order to reduce the amount of fat layered over that exact muscle group. So, like the title says, people believe doing thousands and thousands of sit-ups, crunches, or ab rolls will result in six-pack abs. This myth has its origins alongside the previous myth of burning calories to lose fat.

The thinking with this is you exercise a certain muscle and that muscle starts burning calories, and it just sort of starts burning the calories of the fat which sits layered over it. This is wrong. There is no such thing as spot reduction (well, without surgery). The bigger issue with the idea of spot reduction, though, is it often leads to injury. Fat loss isn't an isolated event; it is a system-wide effect of metabolic changes. If you want to reduce the fat layer over a particular muscle, you gotta feed and work your whole body.

You Have To Spend Hours Per Day Working Out

Whether it's cardio or weights, the common myth is the only way to see real results is to spend at least an hour a day at it. This myth is more of a lifestyle myth than a factual one. It's true if you spend a large amount of time in a particular exercise, you will see significant improvements.

However, it ignores a very important point: recovery. Stressing your body constantly for long periods of time requires you to take adequate time to recover. If you don't allow yourself time to rest and recover, you'll start to break down, get sick, or get injured. Also, the idea of having to spend all that time at the gym or on the road doesn't sound appealing to most middle-aged folks raising a family, working a job, and running a household.

The truth is, and we didn't believe this for a long time – not until we actually put it into practice – you don't have to spend a lot of time working out. You can work out in short, high-intensity sessions, and combine that with occasional longer, low-intensity workouts to get a tremendous benefit to your health.

You Can Tone Your Muscles By Lifting Light Weights

This is similar to the spot reduction myth. The idea behind "toning" is to do a large number of repetitions of light weight. The term "toned" was invented by the fitness industry in the 1980s to sell ridiculous ideas (and fitness VHS tapes) to women. Women became convinced if they lifted heavy, their muscles would look massive and "masculine," and they should, instead, focus on light weight and high repetitions. That method, they said, would lead to "toned muscles."

There is no benefit to doing these kinds of exercises. They don't lead to fat-burning and they don't make you stronger. All they do is waste your time.

We don't care what kind of muscles you have, if they are under layers of fat, you are not toned. So being toned has nothing to do with weights. It has everything to do with what you eat. If you want to lose fat and not get muscular, worry about your diet, not your gym membership.

Stretching is necessary

Not only is stretching not necessary, but current research shows it may actually be harmful to stretch cold muscles. It could lead to injury. The idea behind stretching is to lengthen the muscles, so when you run, lift weights, or whatever, they are already loose and able to take the stress. The idea is based in logic, but has ultimately proven false as a necessity. Stretching itself isn't bad. Yoga is, essentially, long-form stretching and it's fine. Stretching just isn't necessary, and may not be the most efficient way to begin your workout. It doesn't hurt to warm up before you get to the more intense portion of your workout. Jogging for five minutes is more than adequate to get your whole body warmed up and loose.

Lifting Heavy Weights Will Automatically Make You Huge

This is the counterpart of the "toning" myth. The toning myth took off when people convinced women lifting heavy weights would make them huge and masculine. Most women, afraid of not fitting society's concept of feminine beauty, opted for the useless alternative. Building muscle takes time, getting huge takes a lot of time. It doesn't just happen overnight. Lifting heavy is the way you build strength and muscle. Unless you are devoting significant numbers of hours to the pursuit, you won't get huge. You will, however, get stronger, and that's a very good thing.

You Need Sports Drinks/Protein Bars/Supplements

If your health is dependent upon a processed, manufactured food or supplement, you're doing it wrong. There are two main parts to your physical health: your food and your activity. If you are eating a well-formulated ketogenic diet, you won't have a need for those processed, manufactured foods. And if you are exercising outside, in the sun, you will dramatically reduce the need for supplementation, too. Period.

XYZ Exercise Is Ideal For Everyone

Okay, we'll admit there are **two major exceptions** to this myth, but we'll get to them in just a second. Putting those two exceptions aside for just a moment, if someone tells you running or biking or climbing or speed skating is the perfect exercise for everyone, they are wrong. Different people gravitate toward different exercises, because people are different. If you like to run, that doesn't mean it something everyone will like. It also doesn't mean you shouldn't like it if someone else doesn't. Exercise should be enjoyable; if it's not fun, it's not worth it. So find what you like and do it.

Now, for the two exceptions: lifting heavy weights and walking. Those are two things which can benefit every able-bodied person. Lifting heavy keeps your physical self strong and walking for 60 minutes per session can keep your mental health strong.

There are more myths, but these are the big ones. The take-aways for you are: your **diet** controls how much fat your body stores, and you should concentrate on specific kinds of **exercise** to get the most out of them. Oh, and you should enjoy both.

The Ketogenic Athlete podcast interviews guests who have proven, to themselves and those around them, the keto diet can not only bust these exercise myths, but can improve performance and boost PRs in a way glucose tabs and commercial protein bars never could.

Hear their stories at theketogenicathlete.com/category/podcasts

GETTING THE MOST OUT OF YOUR WORKOUTS

Hands down, the best way to get the most out of your workouts is to choose something you enjoy doing. You'll never maximize your workouts if you think of them as punishment or you just don't enjoy them. If you hate running, don't run. If you love swimming, try to incorporate swimming into your routine.

There is a lot of controversy about how one should structure workouts, too. Some people say to alternate between cardio and lifting. Some people say to stick with only one. But what it really comes down to is you and your goals. If you goal is to be a runner, running will be the focal point of your training. If your goal is to improve your body composition, lifting will be front and center.

Regardless of your focus, we are confident lifting heavy stuff is going to help you. Even if you are an endurance-minded athlete, LHS will give you strength and stability to improve your form and increase your energy capacity.

Incorporating all three (lifting heavy stuff, low-intensity aerobics, and high-intensity intervals) will give you fantastic improvements in your exercise efforts. But you want to incorporate them based upon your lifestyle, not the other way around.

So, for example, here's a potential workout schedule:

4 days of LHS 3 days of LIA 2 days of HIIT

That's just an example, and, as you can see, results in nine sessions. Some days would have more than one exercise component. If that won't work for you, that's perfectly okay. Look at your schedule and figure out what matters most to you and where you want to focus your time and effort.

You also must – and we cannot emphasize this enough – you **must** include rest. Whether that means taking days off or having a week of lower intensity, you have to include rest. Getting good sleep is part of that, too. Your body only improves **after** you exercise. So if you don't give it ample time, it won't improve.

The last thing to consider is how often you want to change up your routine. Again, depending on your goals, changing the mixture of the kinds of exercises you do will help you improve. After 4-6 months doing one routine, switch thing up by doing a different lifting schedule or a different weekly schedule.

But, again, regardless of what you choose to do, make it something you enjoy.

PILLAR 3: SLEEP & HYDRATION

The third pillar, sleep & hydration, and the fourth pillar, mindset, might not seem like huge factors when you've already made changes to diet and exercise, but you'd be surprised just how much of an influence they can have on your weight loss efforts.

HYDRATION

Your body is comprised of something around 70% water. So you need to stay hydrated in order to stay healthy.

But there's a saying in the keto world: Drink enough water, but not more.

Your hydration requirements are going to vary, depending on your level of activity, but the best hydration evaluation tool is...well, kinda gross. You're properly hydrated when your urine is straw-yellow to clear.

Yep, you read that right. Take a look before you flush. If your urine is yellow, dark yellow, or brown, you are dehydrated.

However, if your urine is clear, and you are heading to the bathroom every 15 minutes, you are likely over-hydrated. Over-hydration flushes electrolytes, which are critical to the functions of a healthy system.

There's a balance which needs to be struck. And we're talking about **water**, not drinks. **Water** is what you need. Not carbonated water, not soda, not anything other than plain, quality H_2O.

SLEEP

It is not an overstatement to say lack of sleep will destroy all your well-formulated plans. If you aren't getting **at minimum** 6 ½ hours each night, you need to fix something. Lack of sleep causes stress hormones to pervade and you will not see the results you want as quickly as you'd like. But, most importantly, lack of sleep has a direct impact on your cognitive functions. Without sleep, you don't think or react as quickly, and you're far more likely to make bad decisions when you are lacking sleep.

Many fat-adapted people report a lower threshold for required sleep, but this isn't the norm, and it doesn't mean you're doing something wrong if you don't experience the same. And even those people who do sleep less will benefit tremendously from 7 to 8 hours per night of good sleep. So get at least 6 ½ hours per night, and set a goal of 8 hours. You'll feel much better for it.

PILLAR 4: MINDSET

Mindset is the **most important** aspect of a successful keto lifestyle.

In order to maximize your efforts, you have to change the way you think, the way you view the world, and the way you view yourself.

START WITH WHY

When you decide to make a change in your life, a significant, impactful change, you are almost guaranteed to fail unless you ask and answer the single most important question:

Why do you want to do make this change?

One of the reasons that real change, real improvement, fails to take hold in your life is that you don't have this part figured out, and it's the very first thing you should figure out before you do anything else.

This is the fundamental and foundation for your success, so it is not something to be taken lightly. Here are some common **whys**:

I want to lose weight.

I want to look better.

I want to be healthy.

I want to walk my daughter down the aisle at her wedding.

I have a reunion/wedding/event to go to and want to wow my friends (and rivals).

All, some, or none of these may apply to you.

But here's the secret: It doesn't matter **what** your **why** is, but it's crucial you **have** a **why**.

(Actually, there are two secrets. The second is you can have more than one **why**, and you can add and delete them as your progress continues.)

It doesn't matter what your **why** is, because as soon as you assign a value judgment to it, you are invalidating it. If you decide your **why** is dumb, for example, you remove any power it had to drive your efforts and make real change in your life.

Having said that, though, there are two criteria for your **why**, and it's these two things you should use to judge your **why**.

Your **why** must be honest, and it must be relevant.

Your Why Has To Be Honest

This is the biggest stumbling block for a lot of people, because we tend to want to ascribe much more nobler motives to our decisions than we really should. If the most important reason you have for losing fat is because you want to look good in a bathing suit, then be honest about that...and don't pretend it's because you think eating a particular way is better for the environment. Your **why** is the thing which will guide you through the, often, difficult journey of changing your body, mind, and lifestyle. So keep it real, be honest, and own it.

Your Why Has To Be Relevant

This is more subtle, but it has everything to do with your progress. As you move toward your goals, achieve success, and make real change, your **why** will often change. You might start out with a **why** of "I'm tired of not being able to tie my shoes without losing my breath," but once you are tying your shoes like it's no big deal, you might change your **why** to "I want to see that little vein stick out when I flex my bicep." Your **why** will change, and you need to keep it relevant so it has the power to help.

If you keep yourself honest, and you keep a close watch on how your motives change, you are setting up a solid foundation for success.

Why? We're glad you asked.

Because your **why** is your anchor. When you wake up one particular morning feeling sad, or you have a really difficult day at work, or you watch your son suffer through another seizure, your mind will flood with negative thoughts, detrimental ideas, and self-sabotaging plans. If you don't have a solid, honest, relevant **why** in place, you are unlikely to stick with your plan. Chances are, you will just let yourself go, because you will want food to soothe the emotional pain. But if you know why you want what you want, you can combat that negative self-talk with definite, purposeful truths about why you will not allow yourself to succumb to the suck.

Start with **why**, so you can end with success.

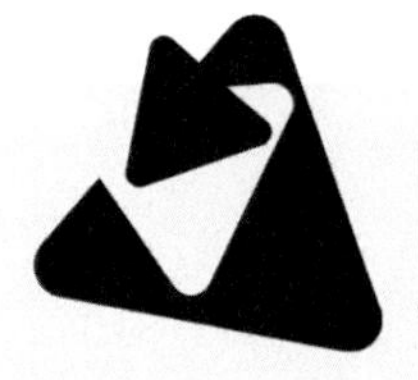

Mindset is a big part of the focus and support offered in the Ketovangelist Unlimited community. If your brain keeps tripping you up, reach out for help at www.ketovangelistunlimited.com

FAT LOSS IS A MENTAL GAME

One of the reasons so many people have trouble losing fat is they don't understand the real cause for their fat gain in the first place. Genetics, of course, plays a huge role in determining how quickly and easily you will become and stay fat. And you can't do anything about your genetics, right?

Well, no. Not exactly.

Stay with us for a minute, so we can explain. Your DNA is made up of four basic building blocks, commonly known as A, G, T, and C (adenine, guanine, thymine, and cytosine), a simple sugar known as dioxyribose, and some phosphate. How these parts get combined and strung together determine things you cannot control, like how tall you are, your eye color, whether or not you have a tail...you get the point.

They also determine things you **can** control, like your willpower, your perseverance, your determination, and your ambition. These are all things corresponding to genetic markers which get turned on and off in certain circumstances. People used to think these things were controlled by DNA and we cannot do anything about them, but latest research shows otherwise.

Current research shows you can, by the choices you make, actually decide which of these genes get activated and which ones get deactivated. For example, you have a gene that we'll call your "mental toughness" gene. This gene activates when you make a difficult, but advantageous, choice. But it deactivates when you cave and decide to take the easy way out. The kicker about this, though, is this gene stays activated until you make a decision which turns it off.

Look into epigenetics if you want to know more. But here's the part we want you to understand. Once you make a tough but necessary decision you know will help you achieve your goals, that gene will stay switched the way you want it. So making the next difficult choice will be easier, because the gene is already switched into the correct position. And the next one, and the next one, and the next one, and pretty soon what you have...is a habit.

This has a tremendous effect on your fat loss efforts, because once you make a series of important, powerful, goal-oriented choices to start or continue down the path to success, you can more easily continue down that path. Making weak or sabotaging choices will make it harder and harder.

We're certain you've experienced this sensation, you just might not know what it was. Your mind is your most powerful fat-loss weapon. If you aren't actively engaging it, every day, you are only extending the struggle.

This is why it's important to give yourself a strict, **non-negotiable** mental boundary.

Addicts who are in recovery are instructed to frame certain things in certain ways. There are lots of different methodologies for this, but they all, basically, come back to two frameworks: acceptable and unacceptable. And it works, so long as you follow it. You must set up your lifestyle to know and understand the things which are acceptable and the things which are unacceptable. And those things **must** remain non-negotiable. You don't get to debate yourself on them, once you've set them up.

For us, bread is non-negotiable. We don't eat it. Ever. In any form. It's not going on our plates, and it's not going in our mouths. Not ever.

The thing is, though, we love bread. Bread is wonderful. And we'll never eat it again, because it's non-negotiable for us. To a beginner, that might sound painful but to us, knowing it's not up for debate, we don't miss it at all.

We have set up our mental boundaries to show ourselves that success is attainable without bread, and bread will cause our failure. It's that simple. And all it took for us to cut it out of our lives was to decide.

One day, we decided we want health more than bread. And that was that.

It started in our minds. And it starts in yours, too. Fat loss is a mental game, and you have to know the rules, the boundaries, and the way to win.

So start today, if you haven't done it already, and decide what is non-negotiable for you. Once you've done that, remove it and don't look back. You will actually be taking deep control of your most basic physical self.

And, don't worry, there are a ton of great food options to fill in for what you remove.

THE SECRET WEAPON TO FAT LOSS

We're about to let you in on a little secret which, if you follow it, will speed your fat loss so much, you might consider it the work of some enchanter. But we can assure you there is no magic involved; it is simple science, logic, and discipline. But before we get to that, allow us a minute to explain where we're coming from.

We're going to take a wild guess and say you've tried multiple times to lose fat, and almost always fail. Of course, there are numerous reasons why we try and fail to achieve fat loss, but we have narrowed down the two primary reasons.

You don't have a goal, or you don't take your goals seriously.

You Don't Have A Goal

Okay, clearly this needs to be explained a bit. Take your **why** (identified in the last section) out for examination. You may have what you **think** is a goal, but chances are all you have is a dream. Most of us have fat loss goals like, "I want to lose 20 pounds." This kind of goal does not follow the good goal guidelines. What are the good goal guidelines? They are SMART goals:

S – Specific M – Measurable A – Actionable R – Realistic T – Timed

A goal should be specific – as detailed as possible. A goal should be measurable, otherwise you have no way of knowing whether or not you've achieved it. A goal should be actionable, because you have to make decisions every day to achieve your goals. A goal should be realistic, otherwise you set yourself up for failure. A goal should be timed, because having a deadline, again, allows for measurability and actionability.

So if we take the "goal" above and compare it to the guidelines for good goals, you see where it falls short. It has no time limit, it isn't specific, and it isn't actionable.

A better goal would be "I will lose at least 4 pounds of fat this month." This goal has all the requirements of a good goal. At the end of the month, you will know whether or not you achieved it. So if you want to improve your fat loss, improve your goals.

Now, for the other primary reason people fail to reach their goals. Get ready; this one might sting a bit...

You Don't Take Your Goals Seriously

No matter how solid and SMART your goals, without this, there is no point at all. Not taking goals seriously is the single biggest cause of failure for every person in the history of humanity, when it comes to fat loss.

Losing fat is really quite simple. You just have to change your habits – what you eat. That's a simple thing. People do it every day. The problem is fat loss is a long-term effort, and cannot be achieved to any degree of satisfaction by making one single change. The change has to happen every day. For some people, it has to happen every hour. When you remove carbs from your diet, you are fighting an addiction. Your body and brain have become dependent upon unhealthy foods and the only way to fix the problem is to remove them (and replace them with healthier ones).

You have to develop different habits. And habits take time. And they take discipline.

So what does this have to do with taking your goals seriously? Everything. Everyday, we choose what foods we shovel into our gobs. It's those choices which determine our success in fat loss. And it's those choices which demand strict respect and unwavering adherence to our goals.

For example, let's say Brian has a goal to lose 10 pounds of fat in two months. Six weeks into the goal period, he's lost seven pounds (just three pounds to go, that's seriously kickass!).

One night, he decides to go out to a restaurant with friends. While there, he is presented with a ton of choices he knows are not conducive to achieving his 10 pound fat loss, and one or two choices which will allow him to continue to achieve his fat loss goal. In the excitement of the moment, because he's with friends and having fun (and perhaps those friends are encouraging him to "treat himself"), Brian decides to indulge and eat whatever he wants.

Brian has just decided he is not serious about his goals. He has decided his fat loss should take a back seat to any possible fun he might have (which he probably could have had, anyway).

If, however, he decided to eat the things he knew were good for his health and fat loss, Brian would be reinforcing the discipline and habits needed to lose the fat. (And Brian's friends should appreciate that. Otherwise, they aren't much like friends.)

In order to achieve your goals, you have to make daily decisions which will lead you to those goals. If you take your goals seriously, you will make the correct decisions, you'll develop the mental discipline, and you'll feed your spirit as well.

So there you have it. These two things can accelerate your fat loss to a point you didn't think possible. It isn't magic, it's logic and discipline.

Try it.

STOP PRETENDING

Living a ketogenic lifestyle requires commitment. There's no way to say it differently because there is no halfway. You must either commit fully to the required plan or you will see absolutely no success. So what does that mean?

It means you cannot pretend. Pretending is when you say (or write) one thing, but your actions don't match your words.

Not pretending means you demonstrate your commitment to your success, by your actions, every day. It means you choose the discomfort of developing new habits over the comfort of the destructive behavior that got you to the place you don't want to be.

One of the most overlooked aspect of choosing a ketogenic lifestyle is the mental effort it requires, not just to make the decision to live a healthier, happier life, but to stick with it when obstacles pop up.

And obstacles will pop up. You have to be able to deal with the difficulties and stay the course. If you don't, you're pretending.

As a real-life example, one of us knows a married mother of three. She's is a go-getter – driven and ambitious to the core. She is also close to 200 pounds overweight. She constantly expresses her desire to lose the fat. Almost weekly, she makes some kind of statement about wanting to get thin. She is exceedingly encouraging to her friends who succeed in their fat loss, and she tells them how she's "so jealous" of their success.

The problem with our friend is, every time she goes out for a girl's night, she eats chips, drinks sugary drinks, chooses the worst foods on the menu, and declares "she deserves it" because of a stressful day, or because she's been good all week (meaning she thinks she made good food choices the previous couple of days), or any other number of reasons.

Her actions do not match her words. She's pretending.

If you say you want to lose fat, but you eat French fries at lunch, you're pretending.

If you say you want to cure type 2 diabetes, but you drink soda, you're pretending.

If you say you want to be strong, but you don't make an effort to lift weights, you're pretending.

If you say you want to get active, but you choose to watch television when you could get up and move, you're pretending.

If you say you want to set a healthy example for your kids, but you smoke, you're pretending.

In all of those examples, the real choice is to choose the actions which fit with what you say. Your actions must match your words. Otherwise, you're pretending, and you're wasting everyone's time. Including your own.

You will find success with your fat loss and your type 2 diabetes when you eat right. For a vast majority, that means a ketogenic diet.

You will find success getting stronger if you lift heavy weights.

You will find success becoming active by getting up and moving, preferably doing something you enjoy.

And, seriously, stop smoking.

There are millions of examples; maybe you've got your own dancing around in your head right now (and that's fantastic). The real point, the real takeaway, is to have a goal and let your actions be consistent with the disciplined determination in achieving that goal. Otherwise, you're pretending.

WINNERS NEVER CHEAT

The question asked more than any other by people starting out on the ketogenic lifestyle is about cheat days. It always intrigues us when the subject comes up, because we're not sure we understand the mindset behind it. To us it sounds like:

"I've decided to change my life, take control, and get healthy...How soon, and how often, can I sabotage those efforts?"

This is not the mindset of a focused, disciplined person, but rather someone who is already resigned to failure. It sounds like us. We've been there. We've made poor decisions, fallen back on old habits and had to start over.

It is what it is. But we don't want you to make the same mistakes. We want you to be successful. And you **cannot** be successful if you're constantly trying to figure out how and when to cheat.

So the answer is: no cheat days.

It's that simple. We're big believers in making things as simple as possible, breaking down decisions to the most fundamental pieces in order to make the best choice. When you first start the ketogenic lifestyle, you'll be faced with choices daily, hourly even, to stay on track or to let the old habits creep in. Thinking about cheat days is self-defeating. The choices you have are, at the most basic point, either: achieve your goals, or indulge in immediate satisfaction. There is no middle ground or compromise. You choose one or the other. You can either eat some crappy food or you can continue to work on becoming the person you want to be: fit, healthy, and awesomer ('cause you're pretty awesome already).

And conquering this choice is a matter of changing your paradigm.

You are **not** trying to lose weight. You are **fighting** an addiction. You have to change how you view this effort – and it **is** an effort at first, fighting the old self in order to allow the new self to grow up.

If someone trying to quit smoking, drinking, or drugs asked, "What about cheat days?" it would be obvious they are not serious about changing. Sticking with the ketogenic lifestyle is exactly the same.

The more you focus on cheat days, the more you focus on not getting the results you want.

So here's some practical advice, learned from many mistakes we made, which we hope you will take to heart. Over the course of the 28-day Kickass Keto challenge, you cannot, **cannot**, consider the idea of cheat days, cheat meals, cheat anything.

You must, absolutely, with pig-headed determination and force of will, **not** stray from the proper ketogenic lifestyle as presented here.

Give yourself these 28 days to stay focused. If you cannot do it, you're not committed. If you can do it, you'll notice a fundamental change in how you view your lifestyle.

Tune Into Positivity

Your mind will believe the truth you feed it. It sees what you focus on.

If you focus on the things you can't have, that deprivation will become the center of your universe.

If you focus on what you want, what you can do, what you can eat, how you will feel, you make the positive feelings the center of your universe. If you focus on your success instead of your old life, the non-keto decisions are going to crop up less and less, because you will only see what you focus on.

So, do yourself a favor, and focus on success. You deserve it, and you ***can*** achieve it. **Because you're kickass!**

We promise you, the first 28 days are absolutely critical. Staying focused on your goal will cause you to change how you view what you used to eat and make you realize how you don't need it, and don't want it, anymore.

But if you fail, realize that you're human. Get up. Restart the clock to Day 1, and get back on track.

After the first 28 days, give yourself 28 more days to continue your focus. **Do not cheat.**

If, after the second set of 28 days, you still feel the urge to cheat, then have a cheat meal. If that cheat meal is satisfying and you love yourself for it afterwards, then remember it and get back on track, reset the clock and go 28 more days eating correctly.

We're willing to bet, though, you will not feel satisfied or happy you indulged. You'll likely feel guilty, gross, and groggy. You might have to deal with your old cravings all over again. That's what cheating does.

But the darker side of cheating is the long-term mental consequences. Just like an alcoholic who has a "cheat drink" is likely to revert to more and more alcohol, a Ketovangelist who has cheat meals/days is likely to fall away.

It's not the ketogenic lifestyle which fails. It's the lack of focus and discipline to stay on track which fails. More often than not, especially if you have no support group, one cheat meal will turn into a cheat day, will turn into a cheat week, will turn into a complete reversion to the unhealthy ways which got you into this mess to begin with.

The absolute, without a doubt, best way to avoid this is to avoid cheats altogether.

So if you have the urge to cheat, even after you notice how much fat you've lost, how your clothes fit different, and how much better you feel, and you've given yourself the crucially important time of two 28-day cycles, have your indulgent meal, snack, whatever.

Hopefully, you'll regret it.

We know we did.

PILLAR 5: COMMUNITY

Doing anything in isolation for a long time is exhausting. As crucial as it is to know your **why**, it's equally important to share your experience with like-minded folks. Having a support network to engage with is a powerful way to stay on track.

Community provides powerful dynamics which benefit participants in many ways, including:

- Belonging – Because our keto lifestyle is strange and confusing to the people in our lives, there are a lot of times when keto living can feel very lonely. Our friends don't understand. Our family doesn't understand. They may try to negate our good mood, or question our decisions, trying to get us to "act normally" when we spend time with them. It's tough, even painful, to experience this. As the *Cheers* theme song goes, "You wanna be where you can see our troubles are all the same..."
- Camaraderie – In life, there will be times when we are discouraged and feeling low, either from outside negative talk, or our own negative thinking. Community lifts us up during these dark moments, reminds us we are not alone, and people do care.
- A Safe Place to Ask Advice – A community can also serve as a brain trust, where you can go for knowledge, advice, and clarification on concepts you may be struggling with, either to understand or enact in your own life.
- Accountability – The right community of people won't let you let yourself down. Many members of our Facebook groups appreciate having a place where they can come for a firm, but gentle, kick in the rear when they know they need some tough love. It's great insurance against the occasional malaise of goal-oriented journeys.

It's about sharing, learning, and giving. It's about community. Talking to someone about your struggles is so powerful, we cannot actually explain how it can help. You need to experience it.

Being a part of an encouraging and accountable community will allow you to stay on track, stay motivated, and stay successful. In any community, there will be different personalities. You'll find someone with whom you connect with and you'll find others with whom you don't. That diversity is crucial to overall success, for all members of the community.

Finding a community in which you can feel safe and free to share, learn, and grow is an absolute necessity.

There are lots of keto communities online which you can join. A word of caution, however: just because they use the term "keto" doesn't mean they are following the same, well-formulated keto diet which you'll find in this book.

Luckily, we have a bunch of communities that we can recommend, because they're ours!

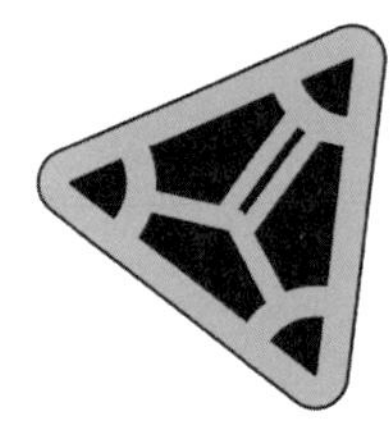

Ketogenic Success Facebook Group

facebook.com/groups/ketogenicsuccess

This is the first stop for general keto knowledge for all levels. Folks can come to the Ketogenic Success group with their keto questions, and know the answers they receive align with the knowledge and science the Ketovangelist team follows.

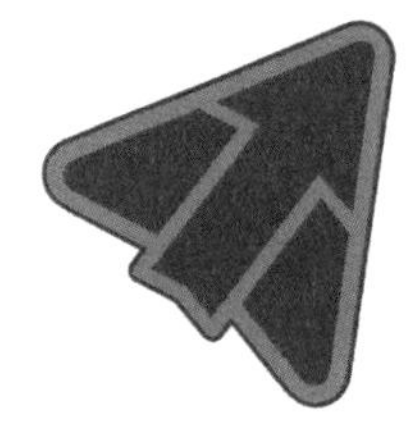

Ketovangelist Kitchen Facebook Group

facebook.com/groups/ketovangelistkitchen

If it's food, it belongs in the kitchen! Folks share recipes, ask for cooking advice, and get a lot of personal responses from Carrie and the admins who know the proper way to make rockstar-level creations in the kitchen!

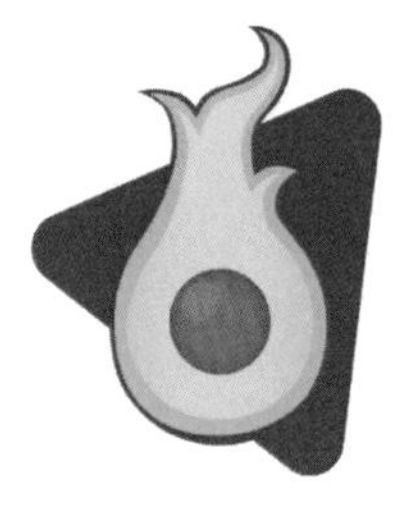

The Ketogenic Athlete Facebook Group

facebook.com/groups/theketogenicathlete

For those folks who are all about using keto to boost up their performance fitness, the Ketogenic Athlete group is focused on fitness, athletics, nutrition maximization, and turning ketones into rocket fuel.

We can vouch for these groups because we run them, and because we have a strong team of admins and moderators to make sure bad information doesn't spread and confuse our members or cause harm.

And, to ensure the groups are full of nothing but the awesomeness you deserve, we also have a strict "No Jerks" policy.

Ketovangelist Unlimited

Ketovangelist Unlimited is an exclusive community dedicated to providing advanced resources to serious Ketovangelists. Carrie, Brian, and Danny Vega, provide thoughtful articles, community challenges, and delicious recipes. KU also has a tight-knit Facebook community featuring amazing support, positivity, and connection with the whole KU membership.

The Facebook group is private to members of www.ketovangelistunlimited.com

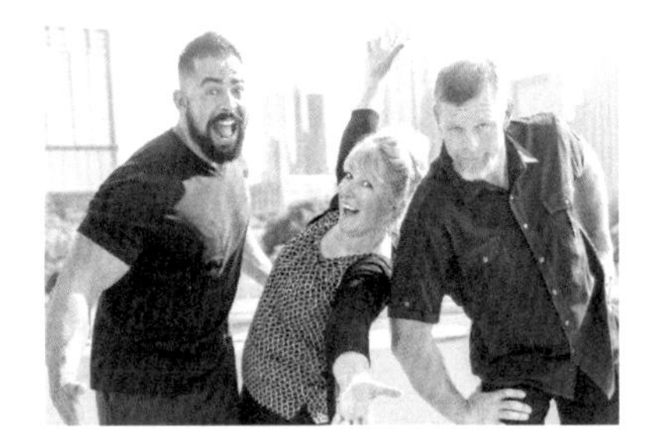

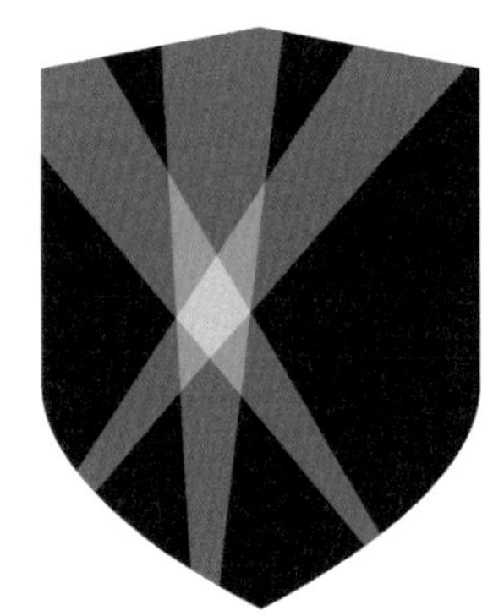

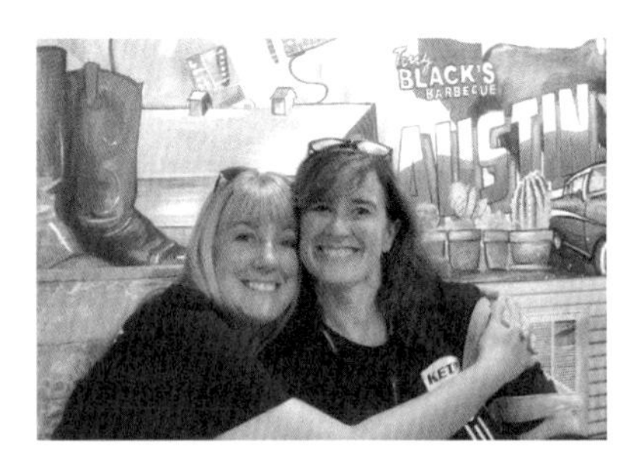

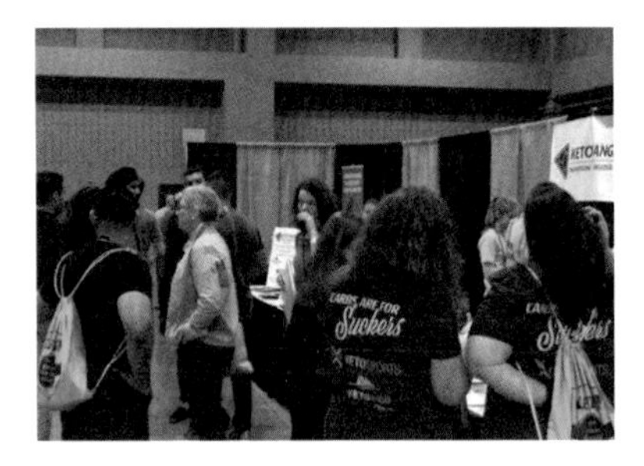

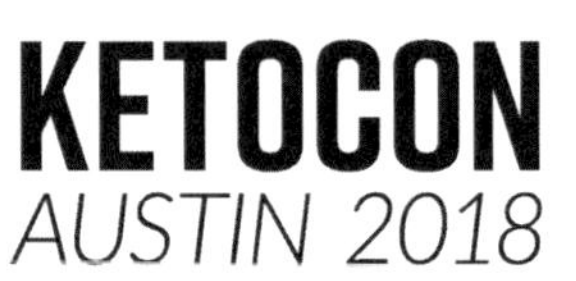

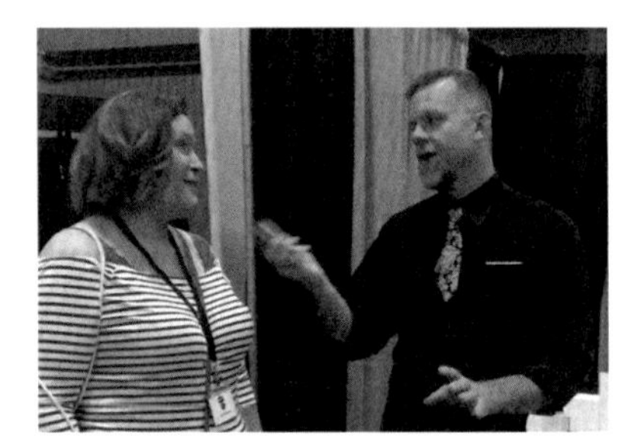

We would also be remiss to mention what a difference it can be to get together, in person, socially, with other Ketovangelists.

In 2017, Brian invited fellow Ketovangelists to Austin, Texas for the biggest keto-focused conference in the United States. Everyone had such an amazing time, people were asking how to buy their tickets for 2018 before they left at the end of the first day!

That's no mistake. It feels **that good** to be surrounded by people who share such as strong bond, and to hear the evidence and validation of our lifestyle presented by amazing experts. And everyone had so much fun talking to the vendors and sampling all the keto-friendly goodies on display. While walking between the booths of nutritious foods and supplements, or demoing ketone breath analyzers, it was easy to imagine the ketogenic diet and lifestyle had already taken over the world!

If you weren't there, don't worry! The Austin conference will be an annual event, and you can learn more, and plan your trip to Austin for the next KetoCon, at ketocon.org.

PART 3: THE KICKASS KETO CHALLENGE

You've reviewed the primary pillars of the challenge, and now it's time to jump in, and leave the SAD life behind!

Four weeks from now, you will have switched from the inflammation-causing carbohydrates which have fueled you for most of your life. The new, fat-burning you will be free from addictive snacks and sugar-level mood shifts, and the fat storage caused by insulin resistance will begin to reverse.

You will want to make sure you have a good belt with at least a few extra holes before you begin! If you don't, no worries, that's no reason not to start today. (You can always reward yourself with a new belt or an updated wardrobe at the end of the challenge!)

The Kickass Keto challenge combines mindset tips, meal plans, fantastic recipes, and suggested fitness routines. We'll offer suggestions on how to tackle prep for the week ahead so you can set yourself up for success.

There are two meal plans to choose from. The first, "Leftovers are Kickass," incorporates leftovers to make your life easier, and is meant for folks who find it impractical to prepare breakfast and dinner seven days a week. The second, "Variety is Kickass," mixes up the menu to tantalize your taste buds with two new keto meals every day.

Whichever plan you follow, you'll get to experience all of the simple, delicious recipes which Carrie crafted for this challenge. You'll save money, because you won't need to keep all those packaged, over-processed snacks around to ward off blood sugar crashes. And you'll get into ketosis in no-time!

Desserts aren't included in the plans, but you can utilize the fat bombs on page 156 if you find yourself in need of some extra fuel. Try to limit these treats to once or twice a week for the best results, and eat them with Meal 3 to let your insulin levels lay low for as much of the day as possible.

PLAN FOR SUCCESS

BEFORE YOU BEGIN

1. Know your why. Your real, honest why. You don't have to tell anyone else what it is. Just own it.

2. Set your goals (three SMART goals). Know how you'll evaluate your success on Day 28.

3. Be ready for success. Believe you can be the person who will succeed and reach your goals!

To help you along the way, this book provides a week-by-week, day-by-day menu, complete with grocery lists and recipes. The idea here is to keep everything simple and easy to follow for as many people as possible. Whether you are a keto veteran or are trying keto for the first time, following these exact steps, day-by-day, will get you into ketosis, keep you in ketosis, and provide you a whole bunch of energy.

The best time to start a ketogenic diet is **right now**. Your 28 day plan starts the day you begin, and work from there. Your days on the plan won't necessarily coincide with the days of the week. If you decide to hold off and start on the next Monday, we highly recommend you begin to cut out starches and sugars with your next meal anyway.

This plan is designed to be delicious, easy to follow, and easy on your budget. Moreover, this plan is designed for your success. Everything is laid out for you; all you have to do is follow the plan. Because we want you to succeed. Because you're awesome!

Clear the Decks

If you can clean the old carbage out of your pantry and fridge, without upsetting any cohabitants, it will help you stay on track. It's much easier to avoid temptation if you'd need to make a run to the store to satisfy a momentary craving.

If you can't toss all the carbage without triggering a mutiny, at least try to rearrange the cabinets so you have a 'keto' shelf as a safe zone, where you won't have to look at the kinds of food you are choosing not to eat any more.

It might also help if one of the carb eaters in the house becomes responsible for buying the kinds of foods they'll be eating, so you can avoid the temptation entirely. We'll leave that negotiation to you, if necessary. Just remember to stay firm, speak with confidence, and stand up for your decision. This is for your health. Re-read the sections on Mindset if you need a quick pep talk.

Shopping List

The recipes are designed to use ingredients multiple times to save on costs, while at the same time mixing up the spices and textures to maximize the variety you will experience.

We also identify things you have purchased already in the 28-day plan which you may not need to buy again. In case you prefer to shop as you need things rather than fill the fridge once per week, we also include the day(s) each ingredient will be needed.

Some of the items you buy will be staples which give you far more than you need for a single recipe. If you are starting with an empty pantry, you may feel like your grocery bill is higher than normal as you fill it with keto staples.

Once you have a few of the basic go-to ingredients, you should see your bill sink lower than ever (and don't forget this plan covers you for every night, so you won't have restaurant bills added on top of grocery bills).

Carrie is also careful to avoid exotic items. Anything in her recipes should be available locally or, at worst, from Amazon.com.

Remember, meat and dairy items can be frozen. The meal plan is organized to maximize the use of produce (fresh veggies) which might go to waste.

Please note this book assumes the plan is being followed by one person and accounts for serving sizes as specified in the recipes. Not everyone has the same appetite, and because you aren't used to eating a ketogenic diet, you won't know how hungry you should expect to be until you're in the middle of it. The typical modern serving size is larger than it needs to be, but we're so used to craving carbs, we don't realize how much we've eaten until we're stuffed. Then, because we burn glucose quickly, we are hungry again later.

Eating keto is very different.

The recipes in this book are sized to give you the leftovers available for Meal 2 the next day or to feed a very hungry person (who can then eat from the Meal 2 Selections list instead). If more than one person will be following this plan, please adjust quantities accordingly.

If you aren't accustomed to eating according to your hunger signals, take care to eat mindfully. If you are used to eating in front of the TV or while working at your desk, try to eat at a table with no distractions until you learn to identify the signal of satiety.

A week or two into the meal plan, you will probably have a good idea of whether your servings are roughly the same size as those recommended in the recipes, and if you need to adjust quantities at all.

If you find yourself ravenous (because perhaps your body has realized there is now high-quality food like it's never known before), keep the extra foods listed under the Meal 2 Selections list around for just-in-case until your hunger regulates.

Prep Ahead

You don't have to prep ahead, but it will definitely make it easier when it comes time to cook (and reduces added prep times for washing and cutting veggies, toasting nuts, etc.).

Here are a few tips:

- Wash, and chop, shred, or slice your produce when you get home from shopping. Wrap veggies in a damp paper towel so they don't dry out, and store them in a plastic bag in the 'fridge.
- If a veggie is called for in multiple recipes, pre-measure out the different quantities ahead of time and chop, dice, whatever the recipe calls for before storing in the fridge.
- Multiple recipes call for riced cauliflower. Many stores now sell riced cauliflower in the fresh produce section, or in the freezer section. Either way, it will cost you more per ounce than whole heads of cauliflower. It's up to you whether the time (or cleaning up the equipment) to rice it yourself is worth the savings. Choose which best suits your lifestyle and priorities. When buying whole cauliflower by weight, keep in mind there will be parts (stem and leaves) you won't use.
- After buying nuts, check which ones need toasting and toast them all together in the oven at once before the week begins.
- Store nuts (and nut flours) in the freezer to keep their oils from oxidizing.
- If you have a bulk store available (such as Costco, Sam's Club, BJs, or whatever your regional version is), get your staples there: bacon, avocado oil (or coconut oil), eggs, cauliflower, meat, and Meal 2 Selections.
- Items which may be more challenging to find will be listed on the prior week's shopping list in case you need to order them from an online supplier. If you find you have to pay shipping, check the whole month's shopping lists to see what else you can order at the same time.
- If you want to be conservative, the shopping lists tell you exactly how much you need for the recipes in the book. If you buy "the next size up" when you grocery shop, ingredients with gray backgrounds remind you to check your fridge for existing supply before you shop. Don't forget to also check your ingredients haven't spoiled!

Staples

Some items will appear over and over again on the shopping lists, and will likely continue to be staples of your keto pantry for a long time. You may want to see which of these you are able to buy in bulk, or which have better pricing available online. Be sure to check out Carrie's Ingredient Guide for all their information (plus links to find them).

http://www.ketovangelistkitchen.com/ingredients-guide/

We worked hard to minimize wasted ingredients, but remember to wrap and freeze the freezable meats and dairy, and we don't recommend buying bags of bulk veggies unless it can't be helped.

MEAL PLAN MENUS

The meal plan is designed to do three things:

1. Provide you with an amazing crash course in just how much YUM a keto diet has in store;
2. Provide you with rich, wholesome food to power your keto journey; and
3. Keep your time in the kitchen and your budget for the groceries to a minimum.

Leftovers vs Variety

Like macro recommendations, meal plans just cannot account for individuality. It's highly improbable someone is going to like **every** recipe in a plan, or **every** ingredient in a recipe. All the same, please give each recipe a fair shot. Rekka doesn't like olives, but **loves** Carrie's Rosemary Olive Cabbage!

Having said that, though, meal plans can be very helpful for diving into a new lifestyle. They remove one of the multiple stressors which come with such a large change. It's impossible to make every person happy with a single meal plan. And we can't know what every person's budget looks like.

But we wanted to give it the best effort we could muster, so this book offers two versions of the meal plan. Both plans use the same 42 recipes, because we don't want you to miss a single delicious bite.

So which should you choose? If you value your time over variety from day-to-day, we recommend you pick the **Leftovers are Kickass** meal plan. This meal plan incorporates leftovers for lunch and dinner, rather than asking you to prepare meals every day of the week.

If you can't imagine eating the same thing two or three days in a row, pick the **Variety is Kickass** meal plan. This meal plan rotates through the recipes before asking you to eat the same meal a second time. It may require preparing meals every night, might fill up your freezer with leftovers, and might cost a tiny bit more at the grocery store to start, but it's all about what helps you stick to the plan! If you do match the days of the week indicated on the menus, it should minimize weekday prep.

Whichever plan you choose, if you're able to, try to "batch cook" some of the more-involved recipes ahead of time. Almost every recipe can be frozen, and those which can't will keep in the fridge for at least a few days so you can enjoy them again.

PRINTABLE PLANNER SHEETS

The following pages contain convenient planners for you to print and fill out with the strategies you have decided will work best for you. It's up to your personal preference and what your goals are. You don't have to fill out every box in the blank trackers.

Put these in a location where they will be the most help to you. If you put them where you'll never look at them, it's just wasted paper!

Remember, it's okay to change up the plan if you get the sense something isn't working for you (once you've given it the old college try, of course).

You may find it helpful to print one habit or fitness planner, fill it out, and photocopy it several times, or print multiple blanks to allow you to try something a little bit different each week.

You'll need:

4 × Blank Habit Tracker

4 × Blank Fitness Tracker

1 ea weekly meal plan and corresponding shopping list (**Leftovers are Kickass** or **Variety is Kickass** per your preferences)

1 × Keto-Friendly Ingredient Guide (or one for work, one for the car, one for the kitchen, etc.)

Because photocopies made from a bound book are never pretty, PDFs of the worksheets are available for you to download and print out at kickassketo.org/kickass-worksheets

WEEKLY HABIT PLAN/TRACKER

Use as many lines of this chart as you need. Be proud of each of your new habits, whether you add one, or one hundred!

Habit For non-daily habits, describe when they will be done. Use a highlighter to pick the days in the right columns.	☑ **Check off each day you repeat your new, healthy habit**						
	Mon	**Tue**	**Wed**	**Thu**	**Fri**	**Sat**	**Sun**
	☐	☐	☐	☐	☐	☐	☐
	☐	☐	☐	☐	☐	☐	☐
	☐	☐	☐	☐	☐	☐	☐
	☐	☐	☐	☐	☐	☐	☐
	☐	☐	☐	☐	☐	☐	☐
	☐	☐	☐	☐	☐	☐	☐
	☐	☐	☐	☐	☐	☐	☐
	☐	☐	☐	☐	☐	☐	☐
	☐	☐	☐	☐	☐	☐	☐
	☐	☐	☐	☐	☐	☐	☐
	☐	☐	☐	☐	☐	☐	☐
	☐	☐	☐	☐	☐	☐	☐
	☐	☐	☐	☐	☐	☐	☐
	☐	☐	☐	☐	☐	☐	☐
	☐	☐	☐	☐	☐	☐	☐

WEEKLY EXERCISE PLAN/TRACKER

	Monday	Tuesday	Wednesday	Thursday	Friday	Saturday	Sunday
Early Morning							
Mid Morning							
Midday							
Afternoon							
Evening							
Notes							

KETO-FRIENDLY INGREDIENT GUIDE

Carbohydrates

- Artichoke
- Arugula
- Asparagus
- Berries
- Bok choy
- Broccoli
- Brussels sprouts
- Lettuce
- Lime
- Mushrooms
- Okra
- Onions
- Parsley
- Peppers
- Cabbage
- Cauliflower
- Celery
- Chia Seeds
- Chicory Greens
- Cucumbers
- Eggplant
- Pumpkin
- Radicchio
- Radish
- Rhubarb
- Scallion
- Shallot
- Snow peas
- Garlic
- Green beans
- Jicama
- Kale
- Leek
- Lemon
- Spinach
- Squash
- Tomato
- Watercress
- Wax beans
- Zucchini

Proteins

- Bass Beef
- Carp
- Chicken
- Crab
- Duck
- Eggs
- Flounder
- Goose
- Halibut
- Lamb
- Mackerel
- Mussels
- Oysters
- Pancetta
- Pepperoni
- Pheasant
- Pork
- Pork rinds
- Quail
- Salami
- Salmon
- Sardines
- Shrimp
- Trout
- Tuna
- Turkey

Fats

- Almonds
- Avocado
- Beef tallow
- Blue cheese
- Brazil nuts
- Butter
- Cheese
- Coconuts
- Cream cheese
- Dark chocolate (≥ 80%)
- Fish oil
- Flax Seeds
- Greek yogurt (plain, full-fat)
- Hazelnuts
- Heavy cream
- Lard
- Macadamia Nuts
- Olive oil
- Pecans
- Pili nuts
- Sour cream
- Sunflower Seeds
- Walnuts

Sweeteners

- Stevia
- Erythritol
- Xylitol

WEEK ONE

THE SECRET OF GETTING AHEAD IS GETTING STARTED.
— MARK TWAIN

This week you begin your journey into better health and happiness. You have made the commitment to your success. It's time to begin.

The Keto Flu

You're going to experience a dramatic shift in energy, but we won't lie to you: the transition may be difficult at first. Your body has been dependent on carbohydrates for fuel for most of your life, and it's going to try to tell you it's suffering without them.

The symptoms of this transition, often called **The Keto Flu**, include:

Headache

Nausea/Loss of Appetite

Disrupted Sleep

Fatigue/Low Energy

Moodiness

Cravings

It sounds weird, but the easiest way through is to embrace the change. You're switching gas tanks on a big rig without the benefit of a mechanic. There are things you can do to minimize the symptoms, but the fact you feel them at all means you're already on the path to becoming fat-fueled. Don't give into the cravings, and you'll emerge on the other side feeling amazing!

Once you burn through your available supply of glucose, your body will start to produce ketones. Because sugar burns so fast, this doesn't take long. If you begin in the morning after a night's sleep, you will likely already have produced ketones.

Until your body transitions to efficiently breaking down fat cells to use for energy, your brain and your muscles will compete for the available ketone supply. Your normal physical performance will likely dip until the transition is complete. Go easy on yourself. You'll know, like a bolt of lightning, when your energy has returned. Until then, try not to expect too much or push yourself too hard.

Additionally, your chronic inflammation will begin to correct itself, and your cells will release retained water. As this water leaves your body, it will flush crucial electrolytes with it. Replacing the electrolytes will help to fight these symptoms, though different people feel relief to different levels.

Sodium – The best source of sodium is sea salt or Himalayan salt. You can take capsules of it, get supplies and make your own capsules, or just take some coarse crystals with water (as you might take acetaminophen).

Magnesium – If you are going to supplement magnesium, use chelated magnesium glycinate. It's trickier to find (hint: Amazon), but the more readily available magnesium citrate and the like will go right through you (if you know what we mean) without replenishing your magnesium.

Potassium – You can combine sodium-free table salts with real salt to supplement potassium, but don't take potassium pills unless directed by your doctor. It's best to get potassium from foods like coffee, avocados, chocolate, and mushrooms, rather than supplement. Luckily, there are plenty of these kinds of foods on the meal plan!

Hydration – Make sure to have water around. Even though you want to flush all that retained water, you need to replace it to flush it more efficiently. We know, the body is weird, right? Keep water available at all times, and drink when thirsty. For the best hydration, we recommend avoiding carbonated beverages such as flavored sparkling water, stevia-sweetened soda, and so on.

MCT Oil or MCT Oil Powder – Medium Chain Triglycerides are ready for use as soon as they enter your system, which means your body, which is a little confused right now, doesn't have to do any extra work to provide them as energy for your muscles. A lot of folks choose to use MCTs throughout their keto life, but they may be especially helpful while you wait to kick into true fat-burning mode. Just a word of caution: go easy. Your body will use what it needs and the rest...well, it won't be stored, which leaves one other outcome. Start with a teaspoon once a day and increase a little at a time until you get used to them and find your sweet spot. If you can't find or afford quality MCT oil sources, Extra Virgin Coconut Oil is the nearest substitute, though it's not as efficient as MCT oil, as it also contains long chain triglycerides.

Exercise Tips for Week One

This week will be the biggest transition for you, and it's totally okay if you don't feel like tackling a structured workout. If all you can manage is a 10- to 15-minute walk, that's great. We'd even advise against doing anything too strenuous, as you'll need your electrolytes to manage the side effects of transitioning from burning glucose to using ketones. If you do anything that leads to sweating, be sure to replace those electrolytes as soon as possible.

If you are normally very active with your fitness, you don't have to stop while you wait to adapt, but take it easy on yourself and don't beat yourself up if you have to drop weight or slow your pace. Your performance will come back stronger than ever when you have fully transitioned to fat burning.

Habit Tracker

Print out the Habit Tracker on page 64 and write in the habits you will try to incorporate this week. Remember, you can start small, such as parking farther away when you are running errands, or saying "no thank you" to the pastry spread in the break room at work. Yes, even things you need to do anyway to become keto are good habits!

If there are any big items you want to work up to, you can add a small habit now to move you in that direction. For example, if you want to eventually run a mile a day, you can add a habit to jog in place for sixty seconds. Eventually you may want to take the stairs up to your job on the sixteenth floor, but for now you can take the stairs up to the second floor and ride the elevator from there.

Every small improvement is a major victory, and that goes for everything you do this week!

The Menu

Choose the meal plan approach that works for you, **Leftovers Are Kickass** for minimal cooking or **Variety Is Kickass** for minimal repeats. At this point, and especially if you have a bare keto pantry to start, you'll have a big shopping trip ahead of you to get started.

If you're not sure which plan to begin with, it's easier to start with the Leftovers plan and switch to the Variety plan after a week, than vice-versa, because the Leftovers plan carries menu items over between weeks.

Note the menus don't specify times of day for your meals, because you will only eat when hungry. If you skip a meal, that's okay!

Get these worksheets as a PDF from kickassketo.org/kickass-worksheets

LEFTOVERS ARE KICKASS – WEEK 1 MEAL PLAN

Week 1 (Day 1-7)	Meal 1	Meal 2 (optional, only if hungry)	Dinner If you choose to eat a fat bomb, eat it with your meal, not as a dessert.
Monday (Day 1)	Hot & Nutty "Cereal" (page 110)	Your choice from Meal 2 Selections (page 124) (Note: this week's menu will leave you with a half avocado, so you can eat that here if you want!)	Chicken & Avocado Salad (page 129)
Tuesday (Day 2)	Baked Cheese & Bacon Breakfast Pie (page 114) (Save 2nd serving in fridge)	Leftover Chicken & Avocado Salad	Steak (page 135) Cilantro Lime Broccoli (page 150)
Wednesday (Day 3)	Leftover Hot & Nutty "Cereal"	Leftover Cilantro Lime Broccoli	Creamy Chicken & Cabbage Casserole (page 128)
Thursday (Day 4)	Leftover Baked Cheese & Bacon Breakfast Pie	Leftover Creamy Chicken & Cab-bage Casserole	Pork Chops (page 134) Hot Bacon & Cabbage Slaw (page 143)
Friday (Day 5)	Coconut Lime Yogurt Supreme (page 112)	Leftover Hot Bacon & Cabbage Slaw	Warm Turkey & Almond Slaw (page 127)
Saturday (Day 6)	Leftover Coconut Lime Yogurt Supreme	Leftover Warm Turkey & Almond Slaw	Salmon (page 136) Avocado Feta Salad (page 154)
Sunday (Day 7)	Ham, Leek & Feta Egg Cups (page 115) (Save 2nd serving in fridge and freeze the rest until called for again)	Leftover Avocado Feta Salad	Prawns with Leeks & Lemon Pepper (page 126)

Print Leftovers Are Kickass – Week 1: Print pages 70 - 73 for menu and shopping list.

LEFTOVERS ARE KICKASS – WEEK 1 SHOPPING LIST

Category	☑	Ingredient	Used in Recipe(s)	Day
Produce	☐	4 oz / 110 g riced cauliflower florets (prepared or process your own)	4 oz for Baked Cheese & Bacon Breakfast Pie	2
	☐	6 scallions (green / spring onions)	2 for Chicken & Avocado Salad 2 for Baked Cheese & Bacon Breakfast Pie 2 for Avocado Feta Salad	1 2 6
	☐	2-4 limes	1 TBSP juice for Chicken & Avocado Salad Zest of 1 + 1 TBSP juice for Cilantro Lime Broccoli Zest of 1 + 4 tsp juice Coconut Lime Yogurt Supreme ½ TBSP juice for Avocado Feta Salad	1 2 5 6
	☐	1 lemon	1 TBSP juice for Prawns with Leeks & Lemon Pepper	7
	☐	20 oz / 565 g leeks	8 oz for Creamy Chicken & Cabbage Casserole 6 oz for Ham, Leek & Feta Egg Cups 6 oz for Prawns with Leeks & Lemon Pepper	3 7 7
	☐	2 ½ oz / 70 g onion	Hot Bacon & Cabbage Slaw	4
	☐	1 English cucumber, quartered and sliced	Avocado Feta Salad	6
	☐	1 ¾ oz / 45 g snow peas	Avocado Feta Salad	6
	☐	fresh rosemary	1 TBSP for Creamy Chicken & Cabbage Casserole 2 tsp for Warm Turkey & Almond Slaw 1 TBSP for Ham, Leek & Feta Egg Cups	3 5 7
	☐	fresh cilantro	1 TBSP for Chicken & Avocado Salad 1 ½ TBSP for Cilantro Lime Broccoli	1 2
	☐	¼ oz / 7 g fresh flat-leaf parsley	Avocado Feta Salad	6
	☐	2 large fresh basil leaves	Avocado Feta Salad	6
	☐	2 avocados	1 for Chicken & Avocado Salad ½ for Avocado Feta Salad	1 6
	☐	1 head of romaine lettuce	To preference for Chicken & Avocado Salad	1
	☐	mixed lettuce greens	To preference for Avocado Feta Salad	6
	☐	11 oz / 310 g broccoli slaw (pre-bagged, try to find without carrots)	5 oz for Cilantro Lime Broccoli 6 oz for Warm Turkey & Almond Slaw	2 5
	☐	15 oz / 425 g cabbage	10 oz for Creamy Chicken & Cabbage Casserole 5 oz for Hot Bacon & Cabbage Slaw	3 4
	☐	4 oz / 110 g mushrooms	4 oz for Prawns with Leeks & Lemon Pepper	7
Meat	☐	7 oz / 200 g bacon	4 oz for Chicken & Avocado Salad 2 oz for Baked Cheese & Bacon Breakfast Pie 1 slice Hot Bacon & Cabbage Slaw	1 2 4

Category	☑	Ingredient	Used in Recipe(s)	Day
Meat (cont'd)	☐	6 oz / 170 g ham	6 oz for Ham, Leek & Feta Egg Cups	7
	☐	1 steak	Steak	2
	☐	1 ½ lb / 680 g Boneless chicken (dark meat is best)	8 oz for Chicken & Avocado Salad 1 lb for Creamy Chicken & Cabbage Casserole	1 3
	☐	1 pork chop	Pork Chops	4
	☐	7 oz / 200 g packet smoked deli turkey, sliced into thin strips	Warm Turkey & Almond Slaw	5
	☐	1 salmon fillet	Salmon	6
	☐	12 oz / 340 g prawns, pre-cooked, de-veined, tail-off	Prawns with Leeks & Lemon Pepper	7
Dairy	☐	12 eggs	3 for Baked Cheese & Bacon Breakfast Pie 9 for Ham, Leek & Feta Egg Cups	2 7
	☐	4 oz / 110 g butter	4 oz for Cilantro Lime Broccoli 2 TBSP for Salmon	2 6
	☐	½ cup / 4 fl oz heavy cream	2 TBSP for Chicken & Avocado Salad 2 TBSP for Baked Cheese & Bacon Breakfast Pie ¼ cup for Creamy Chicken & Cabbage Casserole 1 TBSP for Warm Turkey & Almond Slaw 2 TBSP for Ham, Leek & Feta Egg Cups	1 2 3 5 7
	☐	2 oz / 55 g mozzarella	Baked Cheese & Bacon Breakfast Pie	2
	☐	2 oz / 55 g full fat cottage cheese	Baked Cheese & Bacon Breakfast Pie	2
	☐	1 ½ oz / 45 g cheddar cheese	½ oz for Baked Cheese & Bacon Breakfast Pie 1 oz for Creamy Chicken & Cabbage Casserole	2
	☐	6 oz / 170 g feta cheese	4 oz for Ham, Leek & Feta Egg Cups 2 oz for Avocado Feta Salad	7 6
	☐	2 cup / 16 fl oz plain, full-fat Greek yogurt (NOT non-fat)	1 cup for Coconut Lime Yogurt Supreme ¼ cup for Warm Turkey & Almond Slaw ¼ cup for Avocado Feta Salad ⅓ cup for Prawns with Leeks & Lemon Pepper	5 5 6 7
	☐	½ cup / 4 fl oz sour cream	¼ cup for Chicken & Avocado Salad ¼ cup for Avocado Feta Salad	1 6
	☐	2 oz / 55 g cream cheese	Creamy Chicken & Cabbage Casserole	3
Spices / Pantry	☐	chia seeds	2 TBSP for Hot & Nutty "Cereal"	1
	☐	sunflower seeds	2 TBSP for Hot & Nutty "Cereal"	1
	☐	2 oz / 55 g slivered (not flaked) toasted almonds	2 oz for Warm Turkey & Almond Slaw	5
	☐	unsweetened, shredded coconut	4 TBSP for Hot & Nutty "Cereal"	1
	☐	ground flax seeds	2 TBSP for Hot & Nutty "Cereal"	1

Category	☑	Ingredient	Used in Recipe(s)	Day
Spices / Pantry (cont'd)	☐	1 oz / 30 g flaked coconut	Coconut Lime Yogurt Supreme	5
	☐	1 cup / 8 fl oz canned unsweetened full-fat thick coconut milk	Coconut Lime Yogurt Supreme	5
	☐	almond meal (ground almonds)	4 TBSP for Hot & Nutty "Cereal"	1
	☐	1 ½ oz / 45 g egg white powder	1 oz for Hot & Nutty "Cereal" ½ oz for Coconut Lime Yogurt Supreme	1 5
	☐	vanilla extract	1 tsp for Hot & Nutty "Cereal"	1
	☐	pumpkin pie spice (or cinnamon)	2 tsp for Hot & Nutty "Cereal"	1
	☐	xylitol	2 tsp for Hot & Nutty "Cereal" ½ oz for Hot Bacon & Cabbage Slaw 1 TBSP for Coconut Lime Yogurt Supreme	1 4 5
	☐	dried oregano	1 tsp for Baked Cheese & Bacon Breakfast Pie	2
	☐	sea salt	Too many to list!	1-7
	☐	ground black pepper	Too many to list!	1-7
	☐	celery seed	⅛ tsp for Hot Bacon & Cabbage Slaw	4
	☐	lemon pepper	Prawns with Leeks & Lemon Pepper	7
	☐	½ cup / 4 fl oz avocado oil	2 TBSP for Steak 1 TBSP for Cilantro Lime Broccoli 1 TBSP for Creamy Chicken & Cabbage Casserole 1 TBSP for Warm Turkey & Almond Slaw 1 TBSP for Ham, Leek & Feta Egg Cups 1 TBSP for Prawns with Leeks & Lemon Pepper	2 2 3 5 7 7
	☐	apple cider vinegar	1 ½ tsp for Hot Bacon & Cabbage Slaw ½ TBSP for Avocado Feta Salad	4 7
	☐	white wine vinegar	Warm Turkey & Almond Slaw	5
	☐	guar gum (for week 2, but look around in case you need to order it)	No More Death by Chocolate Frappe	9
	☐	orange extract (for next week, but you may need to order online)	Orange Pecan Brussels & Cabbage	8
	☐	Whatever choices of Meal 2 Selections you want (write in below)	Meal 2 Selections Called for Meal 2 on day 1, then kept as an 'in case' should you eat more than serving suggestions any other day.	1-7

VARIETY IS KICKASS – WEEK 1 MEAL PLAN

Week 1 (Day 1-7)	Meal 1	Meal 2 (optional, only if hungry)	Dinner If you choose to eat a fat bomb, eat it with your meal, not as a dessert.
Monday (Day 1)	Hot & Nutty "Cereal" (page 110)	Handful of dry-roasted Macadamia Nuts (Store extra in freezer)	Chicken & Avocado Salad (page 129)
Tuesday (Day 2)	Baked Cheese & Bacon Breakfast Pie (page 114)	String Cheese	Salmon (page 136) Avocado Feta Salad (page 154)
Wednesday (Day 3)	Vanilla Hazelnut Granola (page 111)	Handful of Almonds (Store extra in freezer)	Creamy Chicken & Cabbage Casserole (page 128)
Thursday (Day 4)	Vanilla Cinnamon Hot Chocolate (page 113)	Hardboiled Egg	Pork Chops (page 134) Hot Bacon & Cabbage Slaw (page 143)
Friday (Day 5)	Coconut Lime Yogurt Supreme (page 112)	Coffee with Heavy Cream	Warm Turkey & Almond Slaw (page 127)
Saturday (Day 6)	Egg & Bacon Salad (page 116)	½ avocado	Steak (page 135) Cilantro Lime Broccoli (page 150)
Sunday (Day 7)	Ham, Leek & Feta Egg Cups (page 115)	Cream cheese-filled celery sticks	Prawns with Leeks & Lemon Pepper (page 126)

Print Variety Is Kickass – Week 1: Print pages 74 - 78 for menu and shopping list.

VARIETY IS KICKASS – WEEK 1 SHOPPING LIST

Category	☑	Ingredient	Used in Recipe(s)	Day
Produce	☐	2 ½ TBSP fresh cilantro	1 TBSP for Chicken & Avocado Salad 1 ½ TBSP for Cilantro Lime Broccoli	1 6
	☐	6 scallions (green / spring onions)	2 for Chicken & Avocado Salad 2 for Baked Cheese & Bacon Breakfast Pie 2 for Avocado Feta Salad	1 2 3
	☐	2-4 limes	1 TBSP juice for Chicken & Avocado Salad ½ TBSP juice for Avocado Feta Salad zest of 1 + 4 tsp juice for Coconut Lime Yogurt Supreme zest of 1 + 1 TBSP juice for Cilantro Lime Broccoli	1 2 4 6
	☐	1 lemon	½ tsp juice for Egg & Bacon Salad 1 TBSP juice for Prawns with Leeks & Lemon Pepper	6 7
	☐	3 avocados	1 for Chicken & Avocado Salad ½ for Avocado Feta Salad ½ for Meal 2	1 2 6
	☐	1 heart of romaine lettuce	To preference for Chicken & Avocado Salad	1
	☐	4 oz / 110 g riced cauliflower florets (prepared or process your own)	Baked Cheese & Bacon Breakfast Pie	2
	☐	¼ oz / 7 g fresh flat-leaf parsley	Avocado Feta Salad	2
	☐	fresh basil	2 large leaves for Avocado Feta Salad	2
	☐	1 bag of mixed lettuce greens	To preference for Avocado Feta Salad	2
	☐	1 English cucumber	Avocado Feta Salad	2
	☐	1 ¾ oz / 50 g snow peas	Avocado Feta Salad	2
	☐	20 oz / 565 g leeks	8 oz for Creamy Chicken & Cabbage Casserole 6 oz for Ham, Leek & Feta Egg Cups 6 oz for Prawns with Leeks & Lemon Pepper	3 4 7
	☐	15 oz / 425 g cabbage	10 oz for Creamy Chicken & Cabbage Casserole 5 oz for Hot Bacon & Cabbage Slaw	3 4
	☐	2 ⅔ TBSP fresh rosemary	1 TBSP for Creamy Chicken & Cabbage Casserole 1 TBSP for Ham, Leek & Feta Egg Cups 2 tsp for Warm Turkey & Almond Slaw	3 7 5
	☐	2 ½ oz / 70 g onion	Hot Bacon & Cabbage Slaw	4
	☐	11 oz / 310g bag of broccoli slaw (try to find one without carrots)	6 oz for Warm Turkey & Almond Slaw 5 oz for Cilantro Lime Broccoli	5 6
	☐	1 small package celery stalks	To preference for Meal 2	7
	☐	4 oz / 110 g mushrooms	Prawns with Leeks & Lemon Pepper	7

Category	☑	Ingredient	Used in Recipe(s)	Day
Meat	☐	11 oz / 310 g bacon	2 oz for Baked Cheese & Bacon Breakfast Pie 4 oz for Chicken & Avocado Salad 1 slice for Hot Bacon & Cabbage Slaw 4 oz for Egg & Bacon Salad	2 1 4 6
	☐	6 oz / 170 g ham	Ham, Leek & Feta Egg Cups	7
	☐	7 oz / 200 g packet smoked deli turkey	Warm Turkey & Almond Slaw	5
	☐	1 ½ lb / 680 g boneless chicken (dark meat is best)	8 oz for Chicken & Avocado Salad 1 lb for Creamy Chicken & Cabbage Casserole	1 3
	☐	1 pork chop	Pork chops	4
	☐	1 steak	Steak	6
	☐	12 oz / 340 g prawns (shrimp) pre-cooked, de-veined, tail-off	Prawns with Leeks & Lemon Pepper	7
	☐	1 salmon fillet	Salmon	2
Dairy	☐	½ cup / 4 fl oz sour cream	¼ cup for Chicken & Avocado Salad ¼ cup for Avocado Feta Salad	1 2
	☐	1 cup / 8 fl oz heavy cream	2 tsp for Chicken & Avocado Salad 2 TBSP for Baked Cheese & Bacon Breakfast Pie ¼ cup for Creamy Chicken & Cabbage Casserole ¼ cup for Vanilla Cinnamon Hot Chocolate 1 TBSP for Warm Turkey & Almond Slaw 2 TBSP for Egg & Bacon Salad 2 TBSP for Ham, Leek & Feta Egg Cups	1 2 3 4 5 6 7
	☐	string cheese	Meal 2	2
	☐	20 eggs	3 for Baked Cheese & Bacon Breakfast Pie 1 egg white for Vanilla Hazelnut Granola 1 for Meal 2 6 for Egg & Bacon Salad 9 for Ham, Leek & Feta Egg Cups	2 3 4 6 7
	☐	2 oz / 55 g mozzarella	Baked Cheese & Bacon Breakfast Pie	2
	☐	2 oz / 55 g full-fat cottage cheese	Baked Cheese & Bacon Breakfast Pie	2
	☐	1 ½ oz / 45 g Cheddar cheese	½ oz for Baked Cheese & Bacon Breakfast Pie 1 oz for Creamy Chicken & Cabbage Casserole	2 3
	☐	2 cup / 16 fl oz plain, full-fat Greek yogurt (NOT non-fat)	¼ cup for Avocado Feta Salad 1 cup for Coconut Lime Yogurt Supreme ¼ cup for Warm Turkey & Almond Slaw ⅓ cup for Prawns with Leeks & Lemon Pepper	2 4 5 7
	☐	8 oz / 225 g (1 stick) butter	1 oz for Salmon 2 oz for Vanilla Hazelnut Granola 1 oz for Egg & Bacon Salad 4 oz for Cilantro Lime Broccoli	2 3 6 6

Category	☑	Ingredient	Used in Recipe(s)	Day
Dairy (cont'd)	☐	2 oz / 55 g cream cheese	Creamy Chicken & Cabbage Casserole To preference for Meal 2	3 7
	☐	6 oz / 170 g feta cheese	2 oz for Avocado Feta Salad 4 oz for Ham, Leek & Feta Egg Cups	2 7
Spices / Pantry	☐	chia seeds	2 TBSP for Hot & Nutty "Cereal"	1
	☐	sunflower seeds	2 TBSP for Hot & Nutty "Cereal"	1
	☐	unsweetened, shredded coconut	4 TBSP for Hot & Nutty "Cereal"	1
	☐	ground flax seeds	2 TBSP for Hot & Nutty "Cereal"	1
	☐	almond meal (ground almonds)	4 TBSP for Hot & Nutty "Cereal"	1
	☐	1 ½ oz / 45 g egg white powder	1 oz for Hot & Nutty "Cereal" ½ oz for Coconut Lime Yogurt Supreme	1 4
	☐	xylitol	2 tsp for Hot & Nutty "Cereal" 3 oz / 85 g for Vanilla Hazelnut Granola 2 TBSP for Vanilla Cinnamon Hot Chocolate 1 TBSP for Coconut Lime Yogurt Supreme ½ oz for Ham, Leek & Feta Egg Cups	1 3 4 5 7
	☐	Macadamia nuts (try for dry roasted, avoid vegetable oils)	Meal 2	1
	☐	almonds	Meal 2	3
	☐	8 oz / 225 g raw hazelnuts	Vanilla Hazelnut Granola	3
	☐	6 oz / 170 g raw slivered almonds	4 oz for Vanilla Hazelnut Granola 2 oz for Warm Turkey & Almond Slaw	3 5
	☐	3 oz / 85 g raw sunflower seeds	Vanilla Hazelnut Granola	3
	☐	sea salt	Too many to list!	1-7
	☐	ground black pepper	Too many to list!	1-7
	☐	dried oregano	1 tsp for Baked Cheese & Bacon Breakfast Pie	2
	☐	lemon pepper	Prawns with Leeks & Lemon Pepper	7
	☐	celery seed	⅛ tsp for Ham, Leek & Feta Egg Cups	7
	☐	ground cinnamon	1 tsp for Vanilla Cinnamon Hot Chocolate	4
	☐	pumpkin pie spice (or cinnamon)	2 tsp of Hot & Nutty "Cereal"	1
	☐	vanilla extract	1 tsp for Hot & Nutty "Cereal" 4 tsp for Vanilla Hazelnut Granola 2 tsp for Vanilla Cinnamon Hot Chocolate	1 3 4
	☐	apple cider vinegar	½ TBSP for Avocado Feta Salad 1 ½ tsp for Hot Bacon & Cabbage Slaw	2 4

Category	☑	Ingredient	Used in Recipe(s)	Day
Spices / Pantry (cont'd)	☐	7 TBSP / 3 ½ fl oz avocado oil	1 TBSP for Creamy Chicken & Cabbage Casserole 1 TBSP for Warm Turkey & Almond Slaw 1 TBSP for Cilantro Lime Broccoli 2 TBSP for Steak 1 TBSP for Prawns with Leeks & Lemon Pepper 1 TBSP for Ham, Leek & Feta Egg Cups	3 5 6 6 7 7
	☐	1 cup / 8 fl oz canned unsweetened full-fat thick coconut milk	Coconut Lime Yogurt Supreme	4
	☐	1 oz / 30 g flaked coconut	Coconut Lime Yogurt Supreme	4
	☐	coffee (ground or cold brew)	Meal 2	4
	☐	white wine vinegar	1 TBSP for Warm Turkey & Almond Slaw	5
	☐	tomato paste	1 TBSP for Egg & Bacon Salad	6
	☐	1 cup / 8 fl oz unsweetened almond milk	Vanilla Cinnamon Hot Chocolate	4
	☐	unsweetened cocoa powder	½ TBSP for Vanilla Cinnamon Hot Chocolate	4
	☐	100% unsweetened chocolate (solid)	Vanilla Cinnamon Hot Chocolate	4
	☐	konjac flour (for next week, but you may need to order online)	¼ tsp for Smoky Creamed Mushrooms	8
	☐	guar gum (for next week, but you may need to order online)	¼ tsp for No More Death by Chocolate Frappe	9
	☐	orange extract (for next week, but you may need to order online)	Orange Pecan Brussels & Cabbage	12

WEEK TWO

*WE SHOULD NOT GIVE UP
AND WE SHOULD NOT ALLOW
THE PROBLEM TO DEFEAT US.
— A. P. J. ABDUL KALAM*

Whew! Last week was...different, right? If you're reading this and you made it to week two, know that your body has a great lead on getting into fat-burning mode. Kickass! Time to forge ahead! The mindset, and possibly also social pressures, are your biggest challenges from here on out. Your body's already figuring out what to do.

Keep up with your electrolytes and hydration. Make sure to adjust your schedule to allow for adequate rest, if you haven't yet.

Exercise for Week Two

If you are feeling more energy, or at least more like yourself, you can begin to add some structured workouts to your routine this week. Alternate core strength with flexibility and cardio, using mostly body weight for your resistance. If you're already walking, try to increase the time and/or distance.

Remember to allow yourself rest days so your muscles can strengthen. The workout breaks down muscle fiber (micro-tears) but the rest days are when your muscles get stronger! There's also evidence that healing muscles burn more calories, so give them the opportunity!

Habit Tracker

If you totally toppled your habit goals for last week, that's awesome! You can add some more, or switch out the ones which didn't take as much focus as you expected. Make sure getting enough sleep is one of your habits if it's traditionally a challenge for you.

The Menu

If you started with one meal plan but want to switch, go for it. Be aware **Leftovers Are Kickass** Week 2 assumes you've got quite a few dishes leftover, so if you were all about **Variety** for Week 1, you might need to do some batch-cooking in order to catch up! Any ingredients you may already have left from Week 1's shopping trip will have a light gray background in the list. Double-check before you shop!

Get these worksheets as a PDF from kickassketo.org/kickass-worksheets

LEFTOVERS ARE KICKASS – WEEK 2 MEAL PLAN

Week 2 (Days 8-14)	Meal 1	Meal 2 (optional, only if hungry)	Dinner If you choose to eat a fat bomb, eat it with your meal, not as a dessert.
Monday (Day 8)	Egg & Bacon Salad (page 116)	Leftover Prawns with Leeks & Lemon Pepper	Bunless Burgers (page 140) Orange Pecan Brussels & Cabbage (page 142)
Tuesday (Day 9)	No More Death by Chocolate Frappe (page 121)	Leftover Orange Pecan Brussels & Cabbage	Double Pork Fried "Rice" (page 130)
Wednesday (Day 10)	Leftover Egg & Bacon Salad	Leftover Double Pork Fried "Rice"	Lamb Chops (page 137) Celery & Cucumber Salad with Herbs (page 147)
Thursday (Day 11)	Vanilla Hazelnut Granola (page 111)	Leftover Celery & Cucumber Salad with Herbs	Montana Hash (page 131)
Friday (Day 12)	Salmon Avocado Omelet (page 118)	Leftover Montana Hash	Chicken (page 139) Mushroom Risotto (page 153)
Saturday (Day 13)	Vanilla Cinnamon Hot Chocolate (page 113)	Leftover Vanilla Hazelnut Granola	Creamy Cajun Sausage Skillet (page 132)
Sunday (Day 14)	Pork Lover's Scramble (page 117)	Leftover Creamy Cajun Sausage Skillet	Pork Shoulder (page 138) Crunchy Winter Slaw (page 155)

Print Leftovers Are Kickass – Week 2: Print pages 80 - 83 for menu and shopping list.

LEFTOVERS ARE KICKASS – WEEK 2 SHOPPING LIST

Category	☑	Ingredient	Used in Recipe(s)	Day
Produce	☐	1 lemon	½ tsp juice for Egg & Bacon Salad 2 TBSP juice for Salmon Avocado Omelet	8 12
	☐	1 orange	zest + juice of ½ for Orange Pecan Brussels & Cabbage	8
	☐	1 avocado	½ for Salmon Avocado Omelet	12
	☐	2 ½ oz / 70 g Brussels sprouts	Orange Pecan Brussels & Cabbage	8
	☐	4 oz / 110 g red pepper	1 ½ oz for Double Pork Fried "Rice" 1 oz for Creamy Cajun Sausage Skillet 1 ½ oz for Crunchy Winter Slaw	9 13
	☐	1 ½ oz / 45 g green pepper	Montana Hash	11
	☐	1 English cucumber	¼ for Celery & Cucumber Salad with Herbs	10
	☐	small package of celery	1 stalk for Celery & Cucumber Salad with Herbs	10
	☐	⅛ oz / 4 g fresh mint	Celery & Cucumber Salad with Herbs	10
	☐	bag of mixed salad greens	½ bag for Celery & Cucumber Salad with Herbs	10
	☐	fresh garlic	2 cloves for Montana Hash	11
	☐	⅝ oz / 15 g fresh flat-leaf parsley	⅛ oz for Celery & Cucumber Salad with Herbs ½ oz for Crunchy Winter Slaw	10
	☐	fresh rosemary	½ TBSP for Mushroom Risotto	12
	☐	1 scallion (green / spring onion)	Salmon Avocado Omelet	12
	☐	7 ½ oz / 210 g cabbage	2 ½ oz for Orange Pecan Brussels & Cabbage 5 oz for Crunchy Winter Slaw	8 14
	☐	18 oz / 510 g riced cauli-flower florets (prepared or process your own)	4 oz for Double Pork Fried "Rice" 5 oz for Montana Hash 5 oz for Mushroom Risotto 4 oz for Creamy Cajun Sausage Skillet	9 11 12 13
	☐	7 ¼ oz / 205 g onion	2 ½ oz for Double Pork Fried "Rice" 1 ¾ oz for Montana Hash 1 oz for Creamy Cajun Sausage Skillet 2 oz for Crunchy Winter Slaw	9 11 13 14
	☐	4 oz / 110 g mushrooms	Mushroom Risotto	12
Meat	☐	¼ lb / 110 g burger patties	1 for Bunless Burger	8
	☐	8 oz / 225 g ground beef (minced beef, aim for 80/20 or fattier)	Montana Hash	11
	☐	1 lamb chop	Lamb Chops	10
	☐	1 pork shoulder	Pork Shoulder	14

Category	☑	Ingredient	Used in Recipe(s)	Day
Meat (cont'd)	☐	10 oz / 285 g ground pork	8 oz for Double Pork Fried "Rice" 2 oz for Pork Lover's Scramble	9 14
	☐	8 oz / 225 g cooked sausage	Creamy Cajun Sausage Skillet	13
	☐	1 skin-on chicken thigh (chicken quarter)	Chicken	12
	☐	1 ½ oz / 45 g smoked salmon / lox, very finely sliced	Salmon Avocado Omelet	12
	☐	8 oz / 225 g bacon	4 oz for Egg & Bacon Salad 3 oz for Double Pork Fried "Rice" 1 ½ oz for Pork Lover's Scramble	8 9 14
	☐	1 oz / 15 g ham	Pork Lover's Scramble	14
Dairy	☐	15 eggs	6 for Egg & Bacon Salad 2 for Double Pork Fried "Rice" 1 white for Vanilla Hazelnut Granola 3 for Salmon Avocado Omelet 3 for Pork Lover's Scramble	8 9 11 12 14
	☐	1 ½ oz / 45 g Parmesan cheese, finely grated	Mushroom Risotto	12
	☐	1 oz / 30 g Cheddar cheese	Montana Hash	11
	☐	7 oz / 200 g butter	1 oz for Egg & Bacon Salad 4 oz for Orange Pecan Brussels & Cabbage 2 oz for Vanilla Hazelnut Granola	8 8 11
	☐	¾ cup / 6 fl oz heavy cream	2 TBSP for Egg & Bacon Salad 2 TBSP for Double Pork Fried "Rice" 3 TBSP for Montana Hash ¼ cup for Vanilla Cinnamon Hot Chocolate 1 TBSP for Pork Lover's Scramble	8 9 11 13 14
	☐	4 oz / 110 g cream cheese	1 oz for Double Pork Fried "Rice" 1 oz for Salmon Avocado Omelet 2 oz for Creamy Cajun Sausage Skillet	9 12 13
Spices / Pantry	☐	½ cup / 4 fl oz beef stock	Montana Hash	11
	☐	¼ cup / 2 fl oz chicken stock	Creamy Cajun Sausage Skillet	13
	☐	1 small can tomato paste	1 TBSP Egg & Bacon Salad 1 TBSP for Montana Hash	8 11
	☐	almond milk	½ cup for No More Death by Chocolate Frappe 1 cup for Vanilla Cinnamon Hot Chocolate	9 13
	☐	coffee (ground or cold brew)	½ cup for No More Death by Chocolate Frappe	8
	☐	cayenne pepper	¼ tsp for Creamy Cajun Sausage Skillet	13
	☐	smoked paprika	½ tsp for Creamy Cajun Sausage Skillet	13

Category	☑	Ingredient	Used in Recipe(s)	Day
Spices / Pantry (cont'd)	☐	onion powder	¼ tsp for Creamy Cajun Sausage Skillet	13
	☐	dried oregano	¼ tsp for Creamy Cajun Sausage Skillet	13
	☐	dried thyme	¼ tsp for Creamy Cajun Sausage Skillet	13
	☐	1 oz / 30 g pecans	Orange Pecan Brussels & Cabbage	8
	☐	8 oz / 225 g raw hazelnuts	Vanilla Hazelnut Granola	11
	☐	Dijon mustard	1 tsp for Montana Hash 2 tsp for Crunchy Winter Slaw	11 14
	☐	unsweetened cocoa powder	3 TBSP for No More Death by Chocolate Frappe ½ TBSP for Vanilla Cinnamon Hot Chocolate	8 13
	☐	1 ½ oz / 45 g 100% un-sweetened chocolate (solid)	1 oz for No More Death by Chocolate Frappe ½ oz for Vanilla Cinnamon Hot Chocolate	8 13
	☐	konjac flour (for next week, but you may need to order online)	¼ tsp for Smoky Creamed Mushrooms	17
	☐	5 ½ oz / 155 g raw slivered almonds	4 oz Vanilla Hazelnut Granola 1 ½ oz for Crunchy Winter Slaw	11 14
	☐	3 oz / 85 g raw sunflower seeds	Vanilla Hazelnut Granola	11
	☐	sea salt	Too many to list!	8-14
	☐	ground black pepper	Too many to list!	8-14
	☐	cinnamon	1 tsp for Vanilla Cinnamon Hot Chocolate	13
	☐	orange extract	Orange Pecan Brussels & Cabbage	8
	☐	vanilla extract	4 tsp for Vanilla Hazelnut Granola 2 tsp for Vanilla Cinnamon Hot Chocolate	11 13
	☐	guar gum	¼ tsp for No More Death by Chocolate Frappe	8
	☐	xylitol	4 TBSP for No More Death by Chocolate Frappe 3 oz for Vanilla Hazelnut Granola 2 TBSP for Vanilla Cinnamon Hot Chocolate 1 TBSP for Crunchy Winter Slaw	8 11 13 14
	☐	9 TBSP / 4 ½ fl oz avocado oil	1 TBSP for Celery & Cucumber Salad with Herbs 1 TBSP for Montana Hash 2 TBSP for Chicken 1 TBSP for Mushroom Risotto 1 TBSP for Creamy Cajun Sausage Skillet 3 TBSP for Crunchy Winter Slaw	10 11 12 12 13 14
	☐	apple cider vinegar	2 TBSP for Crunchy Winter Slaw	14

VARIETY IS KICKASS – WEEK 2 MEAL PLAN

Week 2 (Days 8-14)	Meal 1	Meal 2 (optional, only if hungry)	Dinner If you choose to eat a fat bomb, eat it with your meal, not as a dessert.
Monday (Day 8)	Pork Lover's Scramble (page 117)	Can of Sardines or Salmon	Chicken (page 139) Smoky Creamed Mushrooms (page 144)
Tuesday (Day 9)	No More Death by Chocolate Frappe (page 121)	Leftovers of a Past Meal	Double Pork Fried "Rice" (page 130)
Wednesday (Day 10)	Creamy Lemon Coconut Cereal (page 122)	Sliced Deli Meats	Lamb Chops (page 137) Celery & Cucumber Salad with Herbs (page 147)
Thursday (Day 11)	Coconut Lime Lassi (page 123)	Jerky or Full-fat Greek Yogurt	Montana Hash (page 131)
Friday (Day 12)	Pecan Nutmeg "Oatmeal" (page 120)	Salami Slices	Pork Shoulder (page 138) Orange Pecan Brussels & Cabbage (page 142)
Saturday (Day 13)	Mushroom & Pancetta Frittata (page 119)	Pork Rinds	Creamy Cajun Sausage Skillet (page 132)
Sunday (Day 14)	Salmon Avocado Omelet (page 118)	Handful of Macadamia Nuts	Bunless Burgers (page 140) Crunchy Winter Slaw (page 155)

Print Variety Is Kickass – Week 2: Print pages 84 - 88 for menu and shopping list.

VARIETY IS KICKASS – WEEK 2 SHOPPING LIST

Category	☑	Ingredient	Used in Recipe(s)	Day
Produce	☐	10 oz / 285 g button mushrooms, whole or quartered	6 oz for Smoky Creamed Mushrooms 4 oz for Mushroom & Pancetta Frittata	8 13
	☐	4 oz / 110 g red pepper	1 ½ oz for Double Pork Fried "Rice" 1 oz for Creamy Cajun Sausage Skillet 1 ½ oz for Crunchy Winter Slaw	9 13 14
	☐	1 ½ oz / 45 g green pepper	Montana Hash	11
	☐	2 ½ oz / 70 g Brussels sprouts	Orange Pecan Brussels & Cabbage	12
	☐	1 avocado	½ for Salmon Avocado Omelet	14
	☐	1 orange	zest + juice of ½ for Orange Pecan Brussels & Cabbage	12
	☐	1 lemon	zest + 2 tsp juice for Creamy Lemon Coconut Cereal 2 TBSP juice for Salmon Avocado Omelet	10 14
	☐	1 lime	2 tsp juice for Coconut Lime Lassi	11
	☐	⅛ oz / 4 g fresh mint	Celery & Cucumber Salad with Herbs	10
	☐	fresh garlic	2 cloves for Montana Hash	11
	☐	7 ½ oz / 210 g cabbage	2 ½ oz for Orange Pecan Brussels & Cabbage 5 oz for Crunchy Winter Slaw	12 14
	☐	1 bag mixed lettuce greens	½ bag for Celery & Cucumber Salad with Herbs	10
	☐	English cucumber	¼ for Celery & Cucumber Salad with Herbs	10
	☐	celery	1 stalk for Celery & Cucumber Salad with Herbs	10
	☐	7 ¼ oz / 205 g white onion	2 ½ oz for Double Pork Fried "Rice" 1 ¾ oz for Montana Hash 1 oz for Creamy Cajun Sausage Skillet 2 oz for Crunchy Winter Slaw	9 11 13 14
	☐	scallions (green / spring onions)	1 for Salmon Avocado Omelet	14
	☐	⅝ oz / 15 g fresh flat-leaf parsley	⅛ oz for Celery & Cucumber Salad with Herbs ½ oz for Crunchy Winter Slaw	10 14
	☐	13 oz / 365 g riced cauliflower florets (prepared or process your own)	4 oz for Double Pork Fried "Rice" 5 oz for Montana Hash 4 oz for Creamy Cajun Sausage Skillet	9 11 13
Meat	☐	10 oz / 280 g ground pork	2 oz for Pork Lover's Scramble 8 oz for Double Pork Fried "Rice"	8 9
	☐	8 oz / 225 g ground beef (minced beef)	Montana Hash	11
	☐	¼ lb / 110 g burger patties	1 for Bunless Burgers	14
	☐	1 oz / 30 g ham	Pork Lover's Scramble	8

Category	☑	Ingredient	Used in Recipe(s)	Day
Meat (cont'd)	☐	4 ½ oz / 130 g bacon	1 ½ oz for Pork Lover's Scramble 3 oz for Double Pork Fried "Rice"	8 9
	☐	1 lamb chop	Lamb Chops	10
	☐	1 pork shoulder chop	Pork Shoulder	12
	☐	skin-on chicken thigh (chicken quarter)	Chicken	8
	☐	8 oz / 225 g cooked sausage	Creamy Cajun Sausage Skillet	13
	☐	1 ½ oz / 45 g smoked salm-on / lox, very thinly sliced	Salmon Avocado Omelet	14
	☐	sliced deli meats (your choice, mind the ingredients)	Meal 2	10
	☐	sliced salami	Meal 2	12
	☐	4 oz / 110 g Pancetta	Mushroom & Pancetta Frittata	13
	☐	jerky (mind the ingredients)	Meal 2 (alternative to Greek yogurt)	11
Dairy	☐	16 eggs	3 for Pork Lover's Scramble 2 for Double Pork Fried "Rice" 8 for Mushroom & Pancetta Frittata 3 for Salmon Avocado Omelet	8 9 13 14
	☐	¾ cup / 12 fl oz heavy cream	1 TBSP for Pork Lover's Scramble ¼ cup for Smoky Creamed Mushrooms 2 TBSP for Double Pork Fried "Rice" 3 TBSP for Montana Hash 2 TBSP for Mushroom & Pancetta Frittata	8 8 9 11 13
	☐	4 oz / 110 g cream cheese	1 oz for Double Pork Fried "Rice" 2 oz for Creamy Cajun Sausage Skillet 1 oz for Salmon Avocado Omelet	9 13 14
	☐	¾ oz / 20 g butter	Smoky Creamed Mushrooms	8
	☐	2 oz / 55 g Cheddar cheese	1 oz for Montana Hash 1 oz for Mushroom & Pancetta Frittata	11 13
	☐	2 cups / 16 fl oz plain, full-fat Greek yogurt (NOT non-fat)	1 cup for Creamy Lemon Coconut Cereal Meal 2 (alternative to jerky) ½ cup for Coconut Lime Lassi	10 11 11
Spices / Pantry	☐	½ cup / 4 fl oz chicken stock	¼ cup for Smoky Creamed Mushrooms ¼ cup for Creamy Cajun Sausage Skillet	8 13
	☐	½ cup / 4 fl oz beef stock	½ cup for Montana Hash	11
	☐	1 small can tomato paste	1 TBSP for Montana Hash	11
	☐	Dijon mustard	1 tsp for Montana Hash 2 tsp for Crunchy Winter Slaw	11 14

Category	☑	Ingredient	Used in Recipe(s)	Day
Spices / Pantry (cont'd)	☐	smoked paprika	¼ tsp for Smoky Creamed Mushrooms ½ tsp for Creamy Cajun Sausage Skillet	8 13
	☐	onion powder	¼ tsp for Creamy Cajun Sausage Skillet	13
	☐	dried thyme	¼ tsp for Creamy Cajun Sausage Skillet	13
	☐	cayenne pepper	¼ tsp for Creamy Cajun Sausage Skillet	13
	☐	ground nutmeg	1 tsp for Pecan Nutmeg "Oatmeal"	12
	☐	2 oz / 55 g egg white powder	1 oz for Creamy Lemon Coconut Cereal 1 oz for Pecan Nutmeg "Oatmeal"	10 12
	☐	pecans	6 TBSP for Pecan Nutmeg "Oatmeal" 1 oz for Orange Pecan Brussels & Cabbgage	12 12
	☐	½ cup / 4 fl oz canned unsweetened full-fat thick coconut milk	Coconut Lime Lassi	13
	☐	pork rinds (ingredients should read: "pork, salt")	Meal 2	13
	☐	avocado oil	2 TBSP for Chicken 1 TBSP for Celery & Cucumber Salad with Herbs 1 TBSP for Montana Hash 1 TBSP for Creamy Cajun Sausage Skillet 3 TBSP for Crunchy Winter Slaw	8 10 11 13 14
	☐	apple cider vinegar	2 TBSP for Crunchy Winter Slaw	14
	☐	sea salt	Too many to list!	8-14
	☐	ground black pepper	Too many to list!	8-14
	☐	dried oregano	1 tsp for Mushroom & Pancetta Frittata ¼ tsp for Creamy Cajun Sausage Skillet	13 13
	☐	canned sardines or salmon	Meal 2	8
	☐	1 oz / 30 g 100% unsweet-ened chocolate (solid)	No More Death by Chocolate Frappe	9
	☐	3 TBSP unsweetened cocoa powder	No More Death by Chocolate Frappe	9
	☐	xylitol	4 TBSP for No More Death by Chocolate Frappe 1 TBSP for Creamy Lemon Coconut Cereal 1 TBSP for Coconut Lime Lassi 2 tsp for Pecan Nutmeg "Oatmeal" 1 TBSP for Crunchy Winter Slaw	9 10 11 12 14
	☐	Macadamia nuts	Meal 2	14
	☐	1 ½ oz / 45 g slivered almonds	Crunchy Winter Slaw	14
	☐	sunflower seeds	2 TBSP for Creamy Lemon Coconut Cereal 4 TBSP for Pecan Nutmeg "Oatmeal"	10 12

Category	☑	Ingredient	Used in Recipe(s)	Day
Spices / Pantry (cont'd)	☐	unsweetened, shredded coconut	2 TBSP for Pecan Nutmeg "Oatmeal"	12
	☐	chia seeds	2 TBSP for Creamy Lemon Coconut Cereal 4 TBSP for Pecan Nutmeg "Oatmeal"	10 12
	☐	vanilla extract	1 tsp for Pecan Nutmeg "Oatmeal"	12
	☐	¾ cup / 6 fl oz unsweet-ened almond milk	½ cup for No More Death by Chocolate Frappe ¼ cup for Creamy Lemon Coconut Cereal	9 10
	☐	coffee (ground or cold brew)	½ cup for No More Death by Chocolate Frappe	9
	☐	guar gum	¼ tsp for No More Death by Chocolate Frappe	9
	☐	konjac flour	¼ tsp for Smoky Creamed Mushrooms	8
	☐	orange extract (for next week, but you may need to order online)	Orange Pecan Brussels & Cabbage	8

WEEK THREE

QUALITY IS NOT AN ACT, IT IS A HABIT.
— ARISTOTLE

By this point, many people find themselves free of the symptoms of keto flu. If you are not, that's okay, but take the opportunity to make sure you are following the guidelines in this book without deviation. Remember, every cheat meal is a 'retox' and will set back your progress to becoming truly keto.

Exercise During Week Three

What you do this week largely depends on your energy levels. If you've fully transitioned to fat burning, you may have already found yourself cleaning out the closets in your house or scrubbing the grout in the bathroom just because you didn't know what to do with all that new, excess energy! If that's the case, draft up a fitness plan that can help you burn off that energy and help you sleep even better at night. If you've already been walking for at least an hour a couple times per week (LIA), and strength-training with bodyweight or free weights (LHS), now might be a good time to begin a routine of HIIT. Review some of the suggestions in the section on Fitness to begin experimenting with the type of exercises which you find fun and rewarding.

Habit Tracker

Re-evaluate your habit goals and see if there's anything you want to adjust, replace, or add.

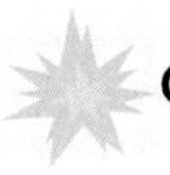

Get these worksheets as a PDF from kickassketo.org/kickass-worksheets

LEFTOVERS ARE KICKASS – WEEK 3 MEAL PLAN

Week 3 (Days 15-21)	Meal 1	Meal 2 (optional, only if hungry)	Dinner If you choose to eat a fat bomb, eat it with your meal, not as a dessert.
Monday (Day 15)	Pecan Nutmeg "Oatmeal" (page 120)	Leftover Crunchy Winter Slaw	Chicken & Avocado Salad (page 129)
Tuesday (Day 16)	Mushroom & Pancetta Frittata (page 119)	Leftover Chicken & Avocado Salad	Salmon (page 136) Avocado Lime Zoodles (page 151)
Wednesday (Day 17)	Coconut Lime Lassi (page 123)	Leftover Avocado Lime Zoodles	Steak (page 135) Smoky Creamed Mushrooms (page 144)
Thursday (Day 18)	Leftover Mushroom & Pancetta Frittata	Leftover Smoky Creamy Mushrooms	Creamy Chicken & Cabbage Casse-role (page 128)
Friday (Day 19)	Creamy Lemon Coconut Cereal (page 122)	Leftover Creamy Chicken & Cabbage Casserole	Chicken (page 139) Bacon Parmesan Brussels Sprouts (page 149)
Saturday (Day 20)	Leftover Ham, Leek & Feta Egg Cups	Leftover Bacon Parmesan Brussels Sprouts	Warm Turkey & Almond Slaw (page 127)
Sunday (Day 21)	Leftover Creamy Lemon Coconut Cereal	Leftover Warm Turkey & Almond Slaw	Prawns with Leeks & Lemon Pepper (page 126)

Print Leftovers Are Kickass – Week 3: Print pages 90 - 93 for menu and shopping list.

LEFTOVERS ARE KICKASS – WEEK 3 SHOPPING LIST

Category	☑	Ingredient	Used in Recipe(s)	Day
Produce	☐	fresh cilantro	1 TBSP for Chicken & Avocado Salad	15
	☐	fresh rosemary	1 TBSP for Creamy Chicken & Cabbage Casserole 2 tsp for Warm Turkey & Almond Slaw	18 20
	☐	1 lemon	zest + 2 tsp juice for Creamy Lemon Coconut Cereal 1 TBSP juice for Prawns with Leeks & Lemon Pepper	19 21
	☐	1-2 limes	1 TBSP juice for Chicken & Avocado Salad ¾ tsp juice for Avocado Lime Zoodles 2 tsp juice for Coconut Lime Lassi	15 16 17
	☐	2 avocados	1 for Chicken & Avocado Salad ½ for Avocado Lime Zoodles	15 16
	☐	1 heart Romaine lettuce	To preference for Chicken & Avocado Salad	15
	☐	14 oz / 400 g button mushrooms, whole or quartered	4 oz for Mushroom & Pancetta Frittata 6 oz for Smoky Creamed Mushrooms 4 oz for Prawns with Leeks & Lemon Pepper	16 17 21
	☐	6 oz / 170 g zucchini	6 oz for Avocado Lime Zoodles	16
	☐	14 oz / 400 g leeks	8 oz for Creamy Chicken & Cabbage Casserole 6 oz for Prawns with Leeks & Lemon Pepper	18 21
	☐	5 oz / 140 g Brussels sprouts (shredded, or process your own)	Bacon Parmesan Brussels Sprouts	19
	☐	6 oz / 170 g bag of broccoli slaw (try to find one without carrots)	6 oz for Warm Turkey & Almond Slaw	20
	☐	10 oz / 285 g cabbage	Creamy Chicken & Cabbage Casserole	18
	☐	scallions (green / spring onion)	2 for Chicken & Avocado Salad ½ for Avocado Lime Zoodles	15 16
Meat	☐	1 ½ lb / 680 g boneless chicken (dark meat is best)	½ lb for Chicken & Avocado Salad 1 lb for for Creamy Chicken & Cabbage Casserole	15 18
	☐	1 skin-on chicken thigh (chicken quarter)	Chicken	19
	☐	1 steak	Steak	17
	☐	4 oz / 110 g Pancetta	Mushroom & Pancetta Frittata	16
	☐	7 oz smoked deli turkey	Warm Turkey & Almond Slaw	20
	☐	1 fillet salmon	Salmon	16
	☐	12 oz / 340 g prawns, pre-cooked, de-veined, tail-off	Prawns with Leeks & Lemon Pepper	21
Meat (cont'd)	☐	6 oz / 170 g bacon	4 oz for Chicken & Avocado Salad 2 oz for Bacon Parmesan Brussels Sprouts	15 19

Category	☑	Ingredient	Used in Recipe(s)	Day
Dairy	☐	¼ cup / 2 fl oz sour cream	Chicken & Avocado Salad	15
	☐	2 cups / 16 fl oz plain, full-fat Greek yogurt (NOT non-fat)	½ cup for Coconut Lime Lassi 1 cup for Creamy Lemon Coconut Cereal ¼ cup for Warm Turkey & Almond Slaw ⅓ cup for Prawns with Leeks & Lemon Pepper	17 19 20 21
	☐	1 ½ cup + 1 TBSP / 12 ½ fl oz heavy cream	2 TBSP for Chicken & Avocado Salad 2 TBSP for Mushroom & Pancetta Frittata 8 TBSP for Smoky Creamed Mushrooms 4 TBSP for Creamy Chicken & Cabbage Casserole 1 TBSP for Warm Turkey & Almond Slaw	15 16 17 18 20
	☐	9 ¾ oz / 275 g butter	1 oz for Salmon 4 oz for Avocado Lime Zoodles ¾ oz for Smoky Creamed Mushrooms 4 oz for Bacon Parmesan Brussels Sprouts	16 16 17 19
	☐	8 eggs	Mushroom & Pancetta Frittata	16
	☐	2 oz / 55 g Cheddar cheese	1 oz for Mushroom & Pancetta Frittata 1 oz for Creamy Chicken & Cabbage Casserole	16 18
	☐	½ oz / 14 g Parmesan cheese, finely grated	Bacon Parmesan Brussels Sprouts	19
	☐	2 oz / 55 g cream cheese	Creamy Chicken & Cabbage Casserole	18
Spices / Pantry	☐	ground nutmeg	1 tsp for Pecan Nutmeg "Oatmeal"	15
	☐	2 oz / 55 g egg white powder	1 oz for Pecan Nutmeg "Oatmeal" 1 oz for Creamy Lemon Coconut Cereal	15 19
	☐	¼ cup / 2 fl oz chicken stock	Smoky Creamed Mushrooms	17
	☐	6 TBSP unsweetened, shredded coconut	2 TBSP for Pecan Nutmeg "Oatmeal" 4 TBSP for Creamy Lemon Coconut Cereal	15 19
	☐	½ cup / 4 fl oz canned unsweetened full-fat thick coconut milk	Coconut Lime Lassi	17
	☐	chia seeds	2 TBSP for Pecan Nutmeg "Oatmeal" 1 TBSP for Creamy Lemon Coconut Cereal	15 19
	☐	sunflower seeds	4 TBSP for Pecan Nutmeg "Oatmeal" 2 TBSP for Creamy Lemon Coconut Cereal	15 19
	☐	2 oz / 55 g slivered almonds	Warm Turkey & Almond Slaw	20
	☐	¼ cup / 2 fl oz almond milk	Creamy Lemon Coconut Cereal	19

Category	☑	Ingredient	Used in Recipe(s)	Day
Spices / Pantry (cont'd)	☐	½ cup / 4 fl oz avocado oil	1 TBSP for Avocado Lime Zoodles 2 TBSP for Steak 1 TBSP for Creamy Chicken & Cabbage Casserole 2 TBSP for Chicken 1 TBSP for Warm Turkey & Almond Slaw 1 TBSP for Prawns with Leeks & Lemon Pepper	16 17 18 19 20 21
	☐	white wine vinegar	1 TBSP for Warm Turkey & Almond Slaw	20
	☐	vanilla extract	1 tsp for Pecan Nutmeg “Oatmeal”	15
	☐	dried oregano	1 tsp for Mushroom & Pancetta Frittata	16
	☐	onion powder	½ tsp for Bacon Parmesan Brussels Sprouts	19
	☐	lemon pepper	Prawns with Leeks & Lemon Pepper	21
	☐	sea salt	Too many to list!	15-21
	☐	ground black pepper	Too many to list!	15-21
	☐	smoked paprika	¾ tsp for Smoky Creamed Mushrooms	17
	☐	xylitol	2 tsp for Pecan Nutmeg “Oatmeal” 1 TBSP for Coconut Lime Lassi 1 TBSP for Creamy Lemon Coconut Cereal	15 17 19
	☐	konjac flour	¼ tsp for Smoky Creamed Mushrooms	17
	☐	pecans	6 tbsp for Pecan Nutmeg “Oatmeal”	15

VARIETY IS KICKASS – WEEK 3 MEAL PLAN

Week 3 (Days 15-21)	Meal 1	Meal 2 (optional, only if hungry)	Dinner If you choose to eat a fat bomb, eat it with your meal, not as a dessert.
Monday (Day 15)	Hot & Nutty "Cereal" (page 110)	String Cheese	Chicken & Avocado Salad (page 129)
Tuesday (Day 16)	Baked Cheese & Bacon Breakfast Pie (page 114)	Handful of Almonds	Salmon (page 136) Avocado Lime Zoodles (page 151)
Wednesday (Day 17)	Vanilla Hazelnut Granola (page 111)	Hardboiled Egg	Creamy Chicken & Cabbage Casserole (page 128)
Thursday (Day 18)	Vanilla Cinnamon Hot Chocolate (page 113)	Decaf Coffee with Heavy Cream	Pork Chops (page 134) Lemon Hazelnut Leeks (page 146)
Friday (Day 19)	Coconut Lime Yogurt Supreme (page 112)	½ avocado	Warm Turkey & Almond Slaw (page 127)
Saturday (Day 20)	Egg & Bacon Salad (page 116)	Cream cheese-filled celery sticks	Steak (page 135) Avocado & Walnut Salad (page 148)
Sunday (Day 21)	Ham, Leek & Feta Egg Cups (page 115)	Can of Sardines or Salmon	Prawns with Leeks & Lemon Pepper (page 126)

Print Variety Is Kickass – Week 3: Print pages 94 - 98 for menu and shopping list.

VARIETY IS KICKASS – WEEK 3 SHOPPING LIST

Category	☑	Ingredient	Used in Recipe(s)	Day
Produce	☐	3 avocados	1 for Chicken & Avocado Salad ½ for Avocado Lime Zoodles ½ for Meal 2 1 for Avocado & Walnut Salad	15 16 19 20
	☐	1-2 limes	1 TBSP juice for Chicken & Avocado Salad ¾ tsp for Avocado Lime Zoodles zest + 4 tsp juice for Coconut Lime Yogurt Supreme	15 16 19
	☐	1-2 lemons	zest + juice of ½ for Lemon Hazelnut Leeks ½ tsp juice for Egg & Bacon Salad 1 TBSP for Prawns With Leeks & Lemon Pepper	18 20 21
	☐	1 heart Romaine lettuce	To preference for Chicken & Avocado Salad	15
	☐	1 hear butter or Bibb lettuce	Avocado & Walnut Salad	20
	☐	4 oz / 110 g riced cauli-flower florets (prepared or process your own)	Baked Cheese & Bacon Breakfast Pie	16
	☐	bag of broccoli slaw (try to find one without carrots)	6 oz for Warm Turkey & Almond Slaw	19
	☐	6 oz / 170 g zucchini	Avocado Lime Zoodles	16
	☐	4 oz / 110 g mushrooms	Prawns with Leeks & Lemon Pepper	21
	☐	fresh cilantro	1 TBSP for Chicken & Avocado Salad	15
	☐	fresh rosemary	1 TBSP for Creamy Chicken & Cabbage Casserole 2 tsp for Warm Turkey & Almond Slaw 1 TBSP for Ham, Leek & Feta Egg Cups	17 19 21
	☐	fresh flat-leaf parsley	1 TBSP for Avocado & Walnut Salad	20
	☐	5 scallions (green / spring onion)	2 for Chicken & Avocado Salad 2 for Baked Cheese & Bacon Breakfast Pie ½ for Avocado Lime Zoodles	15 16 16
	☐	28 oz / 795 g leeks	8 oz for Creamy Chicken & Cabbage Casserole 8 oz for Lemon Hazelnut Leeks 6 oz for Ham, Leek & Feta Egg Cups 6 oz for Prawns with Leeks & Lemon Pepper	17 18 21 21
	☐	10 oz / 280 g cabbage	10 oz for Creamy Chicken & Cabbage Casserole	17
	☐	small package celery	Meal 2	20
Meat	☐	1 ½ lb / 680 g boneless chicken (dark meat is best)	½ lb for Chicken & Avocado Salad 1 lb for Creamy Chicken & Cabbage Casserole	15 17
	☐	1 steak	Steak	20
	☐	1 pork chop	Pork Chops	18
	☐	7 oz / 200 g smoked deli turkey	Warm Turkey & Almond Slaw	19

Category	☑	Ingredient	Used in Recipe(s)	Day
Meat (cont'd)	☐	10 oz / 285 g bacon	4 oz for Chicken & Avocado Salad 2 oz for Baked Cheese & Bacon Breakfast Pie 4 oz for Egg & Bacon Salad	15 16 20
	☐	6 oz / 170 g ham	Ham, Leek & Feta Egg Cups	21
	☐	1 salmon fillet	Salmon	16
	☐	12 oz / 340 g prawns (shrimp) pre-cooked, de-veined, tail-off	Prawns With Leeks & Lemon Pepper	21
	☐	1 can sardines or salmon	Meal 2	21
Dairy	☐	string cheese	Meal 2	15
	☐	2 oz / 55 g mozzarella	Baked Cheese & Bacon Breakfast Pie	16
	☐	4 oz / 110 g feta cheese	Ham, Leek & Feta Egg Cups	21
	☐	1 ½ oz / 45 g Cheddar cheese	½ oz for Baked Cheese & Bacon Breakfast Pie 1 oz for Creamy Chicken & Cabbage Casserole	16 17
	☐	¼ cup / 2 fl oz sour cream	Chicken & Avocado Salad	15
	☐	2 cups / 16 fl oz plain, full-fat Greek yogurt (NOT non-fat)	1 cup for Coconut Lime Yogurt Supreme ¼ cup for Warm Turkey & Almond Slaw ⅓ cup for Prawns With Leeks & Lemon Pepper	19 19 21
	☐	¼ cup / 2 fl oz full fat cottage cheese	Baked Cheese & Bacon Breakfast Pie	16
	☐	2 oz / 55 g cream cheese + extra for Meal 2	2 oz for Creamy Chicken & Cabbage Casserole Meal 2	17 20
	☐	1 cup + 1 TBSP / 8 ½ fl oz heavy cream	2 TBSP for Chicken & Avocado Salad 2 TBSP for Baked Cheese & Bacon Breakfast Pie 4 TBSP for Creamy Chicken & Cabbage Casserole 4 TBSP for Vanilla Cinnamon Hot Chocolate 1 TBSP for Warm Turkey & Almond Slaw 2 TBSP for Egg & Bacon Salad 2 TBSP for Ham, Leek & Feta Egg Cups	15 16 17 18 19 20 21
	☐	12 oz / 340 g butter	2 TBSP for Salmon 4 oz for Avocado Lime Zoodles 2 oz for Vanilla Hazelnut Granola 4 oz for Lemon Hazelnut Leeks 1 oz for Egg & Bacon Salad	16 16 17 18 20
	☐	20 eggs	3 for Baked Cheese & Bacon Breakfast Pie 1 white for Vanilla Hazelnut Granola 1 or 2 for Meal 2 6 for Egg & Bacon Salad 9 for Ham, Leek & Feta Egg Cups	16 17 17 20 21
Spices / Pantry	☐	extra virgin olive oil	4 TBSP for Avocado & Walnut Salad	20
	☐	chia seeds	2 TBSP for Hot & Nutty "Cereal"	15

Category	☑	Ingredient	Used in Recipe(s)	Day
Spices / Pantry (cont'd)	☐	sunflower seeds	2 TBSP for Hot & Nutty "Cereal" 3 oz for Vanilla Hazelnut Granola	15 17
	☐	unsweetened, shredded coconut	4 TBSP for Hot & Nutty "Cereal"	15
	☐	1 oz / 30 g unsweetened, flaked coconut	1 oz for Coconut Lime Yogurt Supreme	19
	☐	1 cup / 8 fl oz canned unsweetened full-fat thick coconut milk	Coconut Lime Yogurt Supreme	19
	☐	unsweetened cocoa powder	½ TBSP for Vanilla Cinnamon Hot Chocolate	18
	☐	½ oz / 15 g 100% unsweet-ened chocolate (solid)	Vanilla Cinnamon Hot Chocolate	18
	☐	ground flax seeds	2 TBSP for Hot & Nutty "Cereal"	15
	☐	almond meal (ground almonds)	4 TBSP for Hot & Nutty "Cereal"	15
	☐	1 cup / 8 fl oz unsweetened almond milk	Vanilla Cinnamon Hot Chocolate	18
	☐	almonds	Meal 2	16
	☐	10 ¾ oz / 305 g raw hazelnuts	8 oz for Vanilla Hazelnut Granola 2 ¾ oz for Lemon Hazelnut Leeks	17 18
	☐	6 oz / 170 g slivered almonds	4 oz for Vanilla Hazelnut Granola 2 oz for Warm Turkey & Almond Slaw	17 19
	☐	2 oz / 55 g shelled walnuts	Avocado & Walnut Salad	20
	☐	sea salt	Too many to list!	15-21
	☐	ground black pepper	Too many to list!	15-21
	☐	pumpkin pie spice (or cinnamon)	2 tsp for Hot & Nutty "Cereal"	15
	☐	ground cinnamon	1 tsp for Vanilla Cinnamon Hot Chocolate	18
	☐	dried oregano	1 tsp for Baked Cheese & Bacon Breakfast Pie ¼ tsp for for Avocado & Walnut Salad	16 20
	☐	lemon pepper	Prawns With Leeks & Lemon Pepper	21
	☐	tomato paste	1 TBSP for Egg & Bacon Salad	20
	☐	coffee (ground or cold brew)	Meal 2	18
	☐	1 ½ oz / 45 g egg white powder	1 oz for Hot & Nutty "Cereal" ½ oz for Coconut Lime Yogurt Supreme	19
	☐	vanilla extract	1 tsp for Hot & Nutty "Cereal" 4 tsp for Vanilla Hazelnut Granola 2 tsp for Vanilla Cinnamon Hot Chocolate	15 17 18

Category	☑	Ingredient	Used in Recipe(s)	Day
Spices / Pantry (cont'd)	☐	xylitol	2 tsp for Hot & Nutty "Cereal" 3 oz for Vanilla Hazelnut Granola 2 TBSP for Vanilla Cinnamon Hot Chocolate 1 TBSP for Coconut Lime Yogurt Supreme 1 ½ TBSP for Avocado & Walnut Salad	15 17 18 19 20
	☐	½ cup / 4 fl oz avocado oil	1 TBSP for Avocado Lime Zoodles 1 TBSP for Creamy Chicken & Cabbage Casserole 1 TBSP for Lemon Hazelnut Leeks 1 TBSP for Warm Turkey & Almond Slaw 2 TBSP for Steak 1 TBSP for Ham, Leek & Feta Egg Cups 1 TBSP for Prawns with Leeks & Lemon Pepper	16 17 18 19 20 21 21
	☐	white wine vinegar	1 TBSP for Warm Turkey & Almond Slaw 2 TBSP for Avocado & Walnut Salad	19 20

WEEK FOUR

THE WILL TO WIN, THE DESIRE TO SUCCEED, THE URGE TO REACH YOUR FULL POTENTIAL... THESE ARE THE KEYS WHICH WILL UNLOCK THE DOOR TO PERSONAL EXCELLENCE.
— CONFUCIUS

Wow, look how far you've come! Seriously. Take a minute to breathe and appreciate what you've accomplished.

By now we hope you have been able to feel the benefits of a ketogenic lifestyle and, like us, you agree carbs have little to offer but poor health and performance. While some folks still may be adjusting to burning fat for fuel, no doubt by now, you are seeing old unhealthy weight gain reverse, and are enjoying the energy and uplifted mood which come with more regulated blood sugar levels (now that they don't spike and dip according to the whims of your food). If you've had chronic pain or other health issues, their symptoms should be easing as well.

Keto really is kickass, and **you're** kickass for sticking with it!

Exercise During Week Four:

As with last week, what you are ready to tackle in terms of fitness will depend a lot on your goals and energy levels. If you haven't tried a HIIT routine yet, give that a shot. Alternate LIA, LHS, and HIIT throughout the week, leaving time for restoration of those exhausted muscle groups.

Habit Tracker

Continue to evaluate your habits with regard to your long-term goals. Revisit the habits you outlined in week one, and add back any which have slipped off your radar.

Remember, self-improvement is a never-ending process. You aren't going to reach a point where you say, "There, I'm perfect now!"

It's a constant process of self-evaluation, goal-mapping, and discovery. Your aim should always be to identify the next practice you can implement to make yourself more kickass than ever.

Get these worksheets as a PDF from kickassketo.org/kickass-worksheets

LEFTOVERS ARE KICKASS – WEEK 4 MEAL PLAN

Week 4 (Days 22-28)	Meal 1	Meal 2 (optional, only if hungry)	Dinner If you choose to eat a fat bomb, eat it with your meal, not as a dessert.
Monday (Day 22)	Leftover Pecan Nutmeg "Oatmeal"	Leftover Prawns with Leeks & Lemon Pepper	Bunless Burgers (page 140) Avocado & Walnut Salad (page 148)
Tuesday (Day 23)	Leftover Ham, Leek & Feta Egg Cups	Leftover Avocado & Walnut Salad	Double Pork Fried "Rice" (page 130)
Wednesday (Day 24)	Leftover Vanilla Hazelnut Granola	Leftover Double Pork Fried "Rice"	Pork Shoulder (page 138) Rosemary Olive Cabbage (page 152)
Thursday (Day 25)	Pork Lover's Scramble (page 117)	Leftover Rosemary Olive Cabbage	Montana Hash (page 131)
Friday (Day 26)	No More Death by Chocolate Frappe (page 121)	Leftover Montana Hash	Lamb Chops (page 137) Leek & Cauliflower Risotto (page 145)
Saturday (Day 27)	Salmon Avocado Omelet (page 118)	Leftover Leek & Cauliflower Risotto	Creamy Cajun Sausage Skillet (page 132)
Sunday (Day 28)	Vanilla Cinnamon Hot Chocolate (page 113)	Leftover Creamy Cajun Sausage Skillet	Pork Chops (page 134) Lemon Hazelnut Leeks (page 146)

Print Leftovers Are Kickass – Week 4: Print pages 100 - 103 for menu and shopping list.

LEFTOVERS ARE KICKASS – WEEK 4 SHOPPING LIST

Category	☑	Ingredient	Used in Recipe(s)	Day
Produce	☐	1 head butter or Bibb lettuce	Avocado & Walnut Salad	22
	☐	fresh flat-leaf parsley	1 TBSP for Avocado & Walnut Salad	22
	☐	fresh chives	A handful for Leek & Cauliflower Risotto	26
	☐	fresh rosemary	1 TBSP for Rosemary Olive Cabbage	24
	☐	2 avocados	1 for for Avocado & Walnut Salad ½ for for Salmon Avocado Omelet	22 27
	☐	1-2 lemons	2 TBSP juice for Salmon Avocado Omelet zest + juice for Lemon Hazelnut Leeks	27 28
	☐	fresh garlic	2 cloves for Montana Hash	25
	☐	5 ¼ oz / 150 g white onion	2 ½ oz for Double Pork Fried “Rice” 1 ¾ oz for Montana Hash 1 oz for Creamy Cajun Sausage Skillet	23 25 27
	☐	1 scallion (green / spring onion)	Salmon Avocado Omelet	27
	☐	16 oz / 455 g leeks	8 oz for Leek & Cauliflower Risotto 8 oz for Lemon Hazelnut Leeks	26 28
	☐	21 oz / 595 g riced cauliflower florets (prepared or process your own)	4 oz for Double Pork Fried “Rice” 5 oz for Montana Hash 8 oz for Leek & Cauliflower Risotto 4 oz for Creamy Cajun Sausage Skillet	23 25 26 27
	☐	5 oz / 140 g cabbage	Rosemary Olive Cabbage	24
	☐	1 ½ oz / 45 g green pepper	1 ½ oz for Montana Hash	25
	☐	1 ½ oz / 45 g red pepper	1 ½ oz for Double Pork Fried “Rice” 1 oz for Creamy Cajun Sausage Skillet	23 27
Meat	☐	¼ lb / 110 g burger patties	1 for Bunless Burgers	22
	☐	1 ½ oz / 45 g smoked salmon / lox, very finely sliced	Salmon Avocado Omelet	27
	☐	cooked sausage	8 oz for Creamy Cajun Sausage Skillet	27
	☐	8 oz / 225 g ground beef (minced beef)	Montana Hash	25
	☐	10 oz / 285 g ground pork	8 oz for Double Pork Fried “Rice” 2 oz for Pork Lover’s Scramble	23 25
	☐	1 pork shoulder chop	Pork Shoulder	24
	☐	1 pork chop	Pork Chops	28
	☐	1 lamb chop	Lamb Chops	26

Category	☑	Ingredient	Used in Recipe(s)	Day
Meat (cont'd)	☐	4 ½ oz / 130 g bacon	3 oz for Double Pork Fried "Rice" 1 ½ oz for Pork Lover's Scramble	23 25
	☐	1 oz / 30 g ham	Pork Lover's Scramble	25
Dairy	☐	8 eggs	2 for Double Pork Fried "Rice" 3 for Pork Lover's Scramble 3 for Salmon Avocado Omelet	23 25 27
	☐	8 oz / 225 g butter	4 oz for Rosemary Olive Cabbage 4 oz for Lemon Hazelnut Leeks	24 28
	☐	¾ cup / 6 fl oz heavy cream	2 TBSP for Double Pork Fried "Rice" 1 TBSP for Pork Lover's Scramble 3 TBSP for Montana Hash 4 TBSP for Vanilla Cinnamon Hot Chocolate	23 25 25 28
	☐	4 oz / 110 g cream cheese	1 oz for Double Pork Fried "Rice" 1 oz for Salmon Avocado Omelet 2 oz for Creamy Cajun Sausage Skillet	23 27 27
	☐	1 oz / 30 g Cheddar cheese	Montana Hash	25
Spices / Pantry	☐	extra virgin olive oil	4 TBSP for Avocado & Walnut Salad	22
	☐	2 oz / 55 g black olives, pitted and chopped	Rosemary Olive Cabbage	24
	☐	small can tomato paste	1 TBSP for Montana Hash	25
	☐	½ cup / 4 fl oz beef stock	Montana Hash	25
	☐	¾ cup / 6 fl oz chicken stock	½ cup for Leek & Cauliflower Risotto ¼ cup for Creamy Cajun Sausage Skillet	26 27
	☐	2 oz / 55 g shelled walnuts	Avocado & Walnut Salad	22
	☐	2 ¾ oz / 80 g hazelnuts	Lemon Hazelnut Leeks	28
	☐	xylitol	1 ½ TBSP for Avocado & Walnut Salad 4 TBSP for No More Death by Chocolate Frappe 2 TBSP for Vanilla Cinnamon Hot Chocolate	22 26 28
	☐	guar gum	¼ tsp for No More Death by Chocolate Frappe	26
	☐	unsweetened cocoa powder	3 TBSP for No More Death by Chocolate Frappe ½ TBSP for Vanilla Cinnamon Hot Chocolate	26 28
	☐	1 ½ oz / 45 g 100% unsweetened chocolate (solid)	1 oz for No More Death by Chocolate Frappe ½ oz for Vanilla Cinnamon Hot Chocolate	26 28
	☐	1 ½ cup / 12 fl oz unsweetened almond milk	½ cup for No More Death by Chocolate Frappe 1 cup for Vanilla Cinnamon Hot Chocolate	26 28
	☐	sea salt	Too many to list!	22-28
	☐	ground black pepper	Too many to list!	22-28

Category	☑	Ingredient	Used in Recipe(s)	Day
Spices / Pantry (cont'd)	☐	dried oregano	¼ tsp for Avocado & Walnut Salad ¼ tsp for Creamy Cajun Sausage Skillet	22 27
	☐	cayenne pepper	¼ tsp for Creamy Cajun Sausage Skillet	27
	☐	smoked paprika	½ tsp for Creamy Cajun Sausage Skillet	27
	☐	onion powder	¼ tsp for Creamy Cajun Sausage Skillet	27
	☐	dried thyme	¼ tsp for Creamy Cajun Sausage Skillet	27
	☐	ground cinnamon	1 tsp for Vanilla Cinnamon Hot Chocolate	28
	☐	vanilla extract	2 tsp for Vanilla Cinnamon Hot Chocolate	28
	☐	Dijon mustard	1 tsp for Montana Hash	25
	☐	¼ cup / 2 fl oz avocado oil	1 TBSP for Montana Hash 1 TBSP for Leek & Cauliflower Risotto 1 TBSP for Creamy Cajun Sausage Skillet 1 TBSP for Lemon Hazelnut Leeks	25 26 27 28
	☐	white wine vinegar	2 TBSP for Avocado & Walnut Salad	22
	☐	coffee (ground or cold brew)	½ cup for No More Death by Chocolate Frappe	26

VARIETY IS KICKASS – WEEK 4 MEAL PLAN

Week 4 (Days 22-28)	Meal 1	Meal 2 (optional, only if hungry)	Dinner If you choose to eat a fat bomb, eat it with your meal, not as a dessert.
Monday (Day 22)	Pork Lover's Scramble (page 117)	Leftovers of a Past Meal	Chicken (page 139) Leek & Cauliflower Risotto (page 145)
Tuesday (Day 23)	No More Death by Chocolate Frappe (page 121)	Sliced Deli Meats	Double Pork Fried "Rice" (page 130)
Wednesday (Day 24)	Creamy Lemon Coconut Cereal (page 122)	Jerky or Full-fat Greek Yogurt	Lamb Chops (page 137) Rosemary Olive Cabbage (page 152)
Thursday (Day 25)	Coconut Lime Lassi (page 123)	Salami Slices	Montana Hash (page 131)
Friday (Day 26)	Pecan Nutmeg "Oatmeal" (page 120)	Pork Rinds	Pork Shoulder (page 138) Bacon Parmesan Brussels Sprouts (page 149)
Saturday (Day 27)	Mushroom & Pancetta Frittata (page 119)	Handful of Macadamia Nuts	Creamy Cajun Sausage Skillet (page 132)
Sunday (Day 28)	Salmon Avocado Omelet (page 118)	String Cheese	Bunless Burgers (page 140) Mushroom Risotto (page 153)

Print Variety Is Kickass – Week 4: Print pages 104 - 107 for menu and shopping list.

VARIETY IS KICKASS – WEEK 4 SHOPPING LIST

Category	☑	Ingredient	Used in Recipe(s)	Day
Produce	☐	8 oz / 225 g leeks	Leek & Cauliflower Risotto	22
	☐	26 oz / 735 g riced cauliflower florets (prepared or process your own)	8 oz for Leek & Cauliflower Risotto 4 oz for Double Pork Fried "Rice" 5 oz for Montana Hash 4 oz for Creamy Cajun Sausage Skillet 5 oz for Mushroom Risotto	22 23 25 27 28
	☐	8 oz / 225 g mushrooms	4 oz for Mushroom & Pancetta Frittata 4 oz for Mushroom Risotto	27 28
	☐	2 ½ oz / 70 g red pepper	1 ½ oz for Double Pork Fried "Rice" 1 oz for Creamy Cajun Sausage Skillet	23 27
	☐	1 ½ oz / 45 g green pepper	Montana Hash	25
	☐	fresh chives	A handful for Leek & Cauliflower Risotto	22
	☐	fresh rosemary	1 TBSP for Rosemary Olive Cabbage ½ TBSP for Mushroom Risotto	24 28
	☐	5 oz / 140 g cabbage	Rosemary Olive Cabbage	24
	☐	5 oz / 140 g Brussels sprouts	Bacon Parmesan Brussels Sprouts	26
	☐	scallion (green / spring onion)	1 for Salmon Avocado Omelet	28
	☐	5 ¼ oz / 150 g white onion	2 ½ oz for Double Pork Fried "Rice" 1 ¾ oz for Montana Hash 1 oz for Creamy Cajun Sausage Skillet	23 25 27
	☐	fresh garlic	2 cloves for Montana Hash	25
	☐	1-2 lemons	zest + 2 tsp juice for Creamy Lemon Coconut Cereal 2 TBSP juice for Salmon Avocado Omelet	24 28
	☐	1 lime	2 tsp juice for Coconut Lime Lassi	25
	☐	1 avocado	½ for Salmon Avocado Omelet	28
Meat	☐	10 oz / 285 g ground pork	2 oz for Pork Lover's Scramble 8 oz for Double Pork Fried "Rice"	22 23
	☐	8 oz / 225 g ground beef (minced beef)	Montana Hash	25
	☐	¼ lb / 110 g burger patties	1 for Bunless Burgers	28
	☐	1 bone-in chicken thigh (chicken quarter)	Chicken	22
	☐	1 oz / 30 g ham	Pork Lover's Scramble	22
	☐	1 pork shoulder chop	Pork Shoulder	26
	☐	8 oz / 225 g cooked sausage	Creamy Cajun Sausage Skillet	27
	☐	1 lamb chop	Lamb Chop	24

Category	☑	Ingredient	Used in Recipe(s)	Day
Meat (cont'd)	☐	sliced deli meat (mind the ingredients)	Meal 2	23
	☐	sliced salami	Meal 2	25
	☐	6 ½ oz / 185 g bacon	1 ½ for Pork Lover's Scramble 3 oz for Double Pork Fried "Rice" 2 oz for Bacon Parmesan Brussels Sprouts	22 23 26
	☐	1 ½ oz / 45 g smoked salmon / lox, very finely sliced	Salmon Avocado Omelet	28
	☐	4 oz / 110 g Pancetta	Mushroom & Pancetta Frittata	27
	☐	jerky (mind the ingredients)	Meal 2 (alternative to Greek yogurt)	24
Dairy	☐	16 eggs	3 for Pork Lover's Scramble 2 for Double Pork Fried "Rice" 8 for Mushroom & Pancetta Frittata 3 for Salmon Avocado Omelet	22 23 27 28
	☐	2 oz / 55 g Parmesan cheese, finely grated	½ oz for Bacon Parmesan Brussels Sprouts 1 ½ oz for Mushroom Risotto	26 28
	☐	½ cup / 4 fl oz canned unsweetened full-fat thick coconut milk	Coconut Lime Lassi	25
	☐	8 oz / 225 g butter	4 oz for Rosemary Olive Cabbage 4 oz for Bacon Parmesan Brussels Sprouts	24 26
	☐	½ cup / 4 fl oz heavy cream	1 TBSP for Pork Lover's Scramble 2 TBSP for Double Pork Fried "Rice" 3 TBSP for Montana Hash 2 TBSP for Mushroom & Pancetta Frittata	22 23 25 27
	☐	4 oz / 110 g cream cheese	1 oz for Double Pork Fried "Rice" 2 oz for Creamy Cajun Sausage Skillet 1 oz for Salmon Avocado Omelet	23 27 28
	☐	2 cups / 16 fl oz plain, full-fat Greek yogurt (NOT non-fat)	Meal 2 (alternative to Jerky) 1 cup for Creamy Lemon Coconut Cereal ½ cup for Coconut Lime Lassi	24 24 25
	☐	2 oz / 55 g Cheddar cheese	1 oz for Montana Hash 1 oz for Mushroom & Pancetta Frittata	25 27
	☐	string cheese	Meal 2	28
Spices / Pantry	☐	2 oz / 55 g black olives, pitted and finely chopped	Rosemary Olive Cabbage	24
	☐	small can tomato paste	1 TBSP for Montana Hash	25
	☐	sea salt	Too many to list!	22-28
	☐	ground black pepper	Too many to list!	22-28
	☐	dried oregano	1 tsp for Mushroom & Pancetta Frittata ¼ tsp for Creamy Cajun Sausage Skillet	27 27

Category	☑	Ingredient	Used in Recipe(s)	Day
Spices / Pantry (cont'd)	☐	dried thyme	¼ tsp for Creamy Cajun Sausage Skillet	27
	☐	onion powder	½ tsp for Bacon Parmesan Brussels Sprouts ¼ tsp for Creamy Cajun Sausage Skillet	26 27
	☐	cayenne pepper	¼ tsp for Creamy Cajun Sausage Skillet	27
	☐	smoked paprika	½ tsp for Creamy Cajun Sausage Skillet	27
	☐	ground nutmeg	1 tsp for Pecan Nutmeg "Oatmeal"	26
	☐	vanilla extract	1 tsp for Pecan Nutmeg "Oatmeal"	26
	☐	egg white powder	1 oz for Creamy Lemon Coconut Cereal 1 oz for Pecan Nutmeg "Oatmeal"	24 26
	☐	⅜ cup / 3 fl oz avocado oil	2 TBSP for Chicken 1 TBSP for Leek & Cauliflower Risotto 1 TBSP for Montana Hash 1 TBSP for Creamy Cajun Sausage Skillet 1 TBSP for Mushroom Risotto	22 22 25 27 28
	☐	Dijon mustard	1 tsp for Montana Hash	25
	☐	½ cup / 4 fl oz beef stock	Montana Hash	25
	☐	¾ cup / 6 fl oz chicken stock	½ cup for Leek & Cauliflower Risotto ¼ cup for Creamy Cajun Sausage Skillet	22 27
	☐	pork rinds (ingredients should read: "pork, salt")	Meal 2	26
	☐	¾ cup / 6 fl oz almond milk	½ cup for No More Death by Chocolate Frappe ¼ cup for Creamy Lemon Coconut Cereal	23 24
	☐	2 oz / 55 g sunflower seeds	1 oz for Creamy Lemon Coconut Cereal 1 oz for Pecan Nutmeg "Oatmeal"	24 26
	☐	2 oz / 55 g chia seeds	1 oz for Creamy Lemon Coconut Cereal 1 oz for Pecan Nutmeg "Oatmeal"	24 26
	☐	pecans	6 TBSP for Pecan Nutmeg "Oatmeal"	26
	☐	Macadamia nuts	Meal 2	27
	☐	2 oz / 55 g unsweetened, shredded coconut	1 oz for Creamy Lemon Coconut Cereal 1 oz for Pecan Nutmeg "Oatmeal"	24 26
	☐	coffee (ground or cold brew)	½ cup for No More Death by Chocolate Frappe	23
	☐	unsweetened cocoa powder	3 TBSP for No More Death by Chocolate Frappe	23
	☐	1 oz / 30 g 100% unsweet-ened chocolate (solid)	No More Death by Chocolate Frappe	23
	☐	xylitol	4 TBSP for No More Death by Chocolate Frappe 1 TBSP for Creamy Lemon Coconut Cereal 1 TBSP for Coconut Lime Lassi 2 tsp for Pecan Nutmeg "Oatmeal"	23 24 25 26
	☐	guar gum	¼ tsp for No More Death by Chocolate Frappe	23

PART 4: THE RECIPES

MEAL 1

BREAKFAST IS THE MOST IMPORTANT MEAL OF THE DAY. — EVERY SAD NUTRITION EXPERT AND MOM, EVER

The thing is, they're not wrong. The difference is in the timing.

Most of us understand that the word "breakfast" comes from "to break the fast." And by its classical definition, yes, breakfast is the most important meal of the day. While you fast, which we most readily do overnight, your body can do some serious healing. When we break our fast, we reward all that healing with raw materials for continued health improvement.

Unfortunately in our modern society, "breakfast" has come to mean something more along the lines of "that bowl of cereal or bagel you wolf down on your way to wherever you're already running ten minutes late to reach and oh yeah if you did the shopping maybe there's an orange or apple."

It's a rushed meal, and by SAD guidelines, it's low-fat, grain-based, and high-sugar. Not to mention highly processed.

There's a reason high-performers tend to be the type to grab a coffee on their way out the door for their morning commute: **you don't necessarily need to eat first thing in the morning**, and you definitely don't need to fuel up on carbage.

So, in this book, we use the term "Meal 1" to indicate food with which you break your fast, just to remove ourselves from the expectation it'll come first thing in the morning. Break your fast with a Meal 1 recipe at whatever point in the day your body signals it's truly hungry.

HOT & NUTTY "CEREAL"

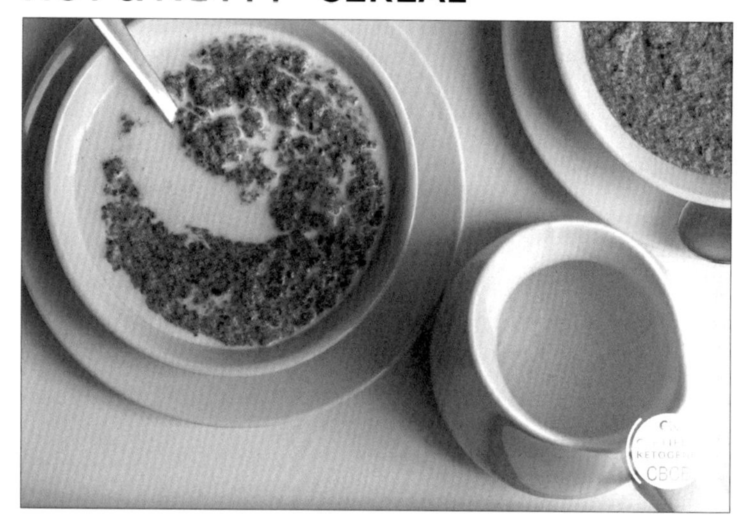

Servings:
2
Category:
Meal 1
Prep time:
5 minutes
Cook time:
2 minutes
Total time:
7 minutes
CertifiedKetogenic.com **Rating:**
Certified Ketogenic

WHAT YOU NEED

2 TBSP chia seeds

2 TBSP sunflower seeds

4 TBSP unsweetened, shredded coconut

2 TBSP ground flax seeds

4 TBSP almond meal (ground almonds)

2 tsp pumpkin pie spice (or cinnamon if you don't have pumpkin pie spice)

1 oz / 30g egg white powder

1 cup / 8 fl oz boiling water

1 tsp vanilla extract

2 tsp xylitol or erythritol (or more to taste)

WHAT YOU DO

1. Place chia seeds, sunflower seeds, and coconut in a coffee grinder and grind until fine. (If you use a high-powered blender, be careful you don't end up with a paste!)
2. Pour ground mix into a bowl, add ground flax seeds, almond meal, spice and egg white powder and mix well until completely blended.
3. Add cup of boiling water and stir well. Leave to sit for one minute to thicken. Stir and add more boiling water if you prefer a runnier cereal.
4. Add vanilla extract, and xylitol or erythritol to sweeten to taste, and serve with heavy cream if the mood takes you. Which it probably will.

NOTES

- For one serving, use half the mix and add ½ cup / 4 fl oz boiling water.

VANILLA HAZELNUT GRANOLA

Servings:
8 × 1 oz / 30 g servings
Category:
Meal 1
Prep time:
10 minutes
Cook time:
50 minutes
Total time:
1 hour
CertifiedKetogenic.com **Rating:**
Certified Ketogenic

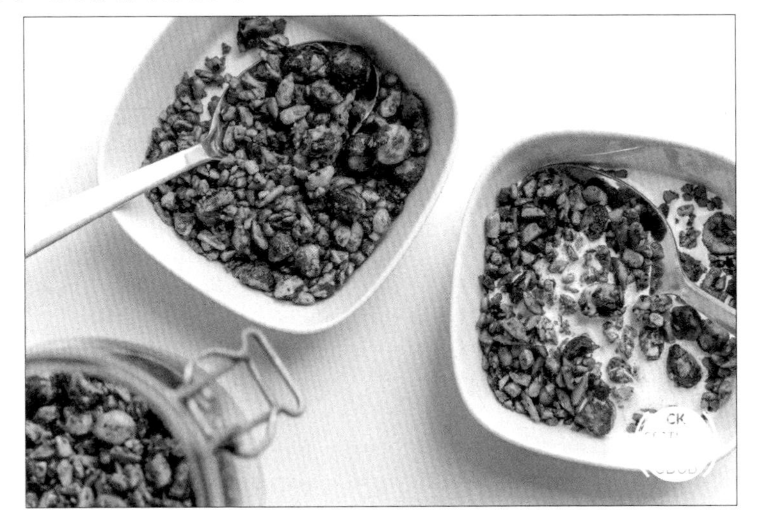

WHAT YOU NEED

2 oz / 55 g butter

3 oz / 85 g xylitol or erythritol

¼ tsp sea salt

4 tsp vanilla extract

1 egg white, whisked until frothy

8 oz / 225 g raw hazelnuts, roughly chopped

4 oz / 110 g raw slivered almonds, roughly chopped

3 oz / 85 g raw sunflower seeds, roughly chopped

WHAT YOU DO

1. Gently warm the butter, xylitol or erythritol, sea salt and vanilla extract in a small pan, just until completely melted.
2. Pour melted butter mixture into a large bowl and quickly whisk in the frothy egg white.
3. Add the roughly chopped hazelnuts, almonds, and sunflower seeds to the bowl and mix well until all the nuts are completely coated.
4. Spread the nuts evenly on a baking tray (preferably one that has sides) and bake in the center of the oven at 300F for 50 minutes until golden brown, stirring well and then re-spreading evenly on the tray about every 10 minutes.
5. After 50 minutes, remove from oven and leave to cool completely on the baking sheet.
6. Once the granola is cold, store in an airtight jar.
7. Serve with heavy cream or a 1:1 mix of heavy cream and water if you prefer a thinner liquid on your granola.

COCONUT LIME YOGURT SUPREME

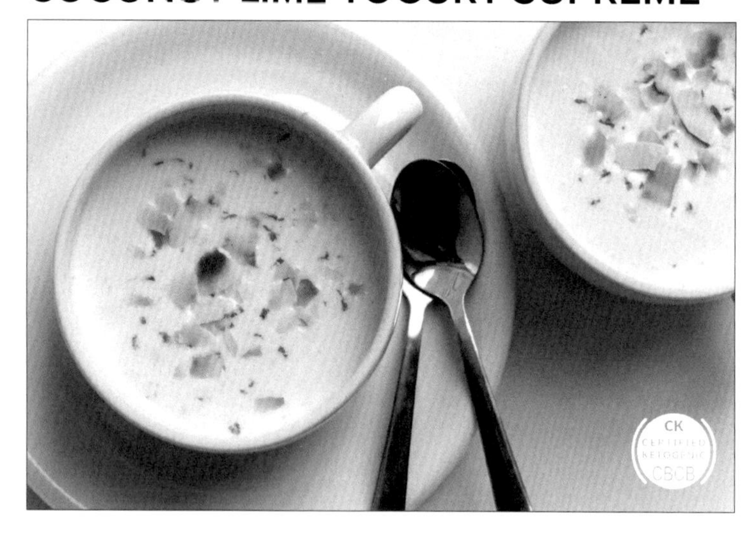

Servings:
2
Category:
Meal 1
Prep time:
5 minutes
Cook time:
1 minute
Total time:
6 minutes
CertifiedKetogenic.com **Rating:**
Certified Ketogenic

WHAT YOU NEED

1 cup / 8 fl oz plain, unsweetened full-fat Greek yogurt

1 cup / 8 fl oz canned unsweetened full-fat thick coconut milk

½ oz / 15 g egg white powder

zest of one lime

4 tsp lime juice (from the lime you just zested)

1 TBSP xylitol or erythritol

1 oz / 30 g flaked coconut

WHAT YOU DO

1. In a bowl, mix the yogurt, thick coconut milk, egg white powder, lime zest and juice, and xylitol or erythritol together well, until it is smooth and completely mixed.
2. Toast the flaked coconut until the broiler (grill) just until gently toasted – this will happen very fast. Do not walk away otherwise you will have burnt coconut.
3. Gently stir the toasted flaked coconut in to the yogurt.
4. Store in an airtight container in the 'fridge.

VANILLA CINNAMON HOT CHOCOLATE

Servings:
1
Category:
Meal 1
Prep time:
2 minutes
Cook time:
5 minutes
Total time:
7 minutes
CertifiedKetogenic.com **Rating:**
Certified Ketogenic

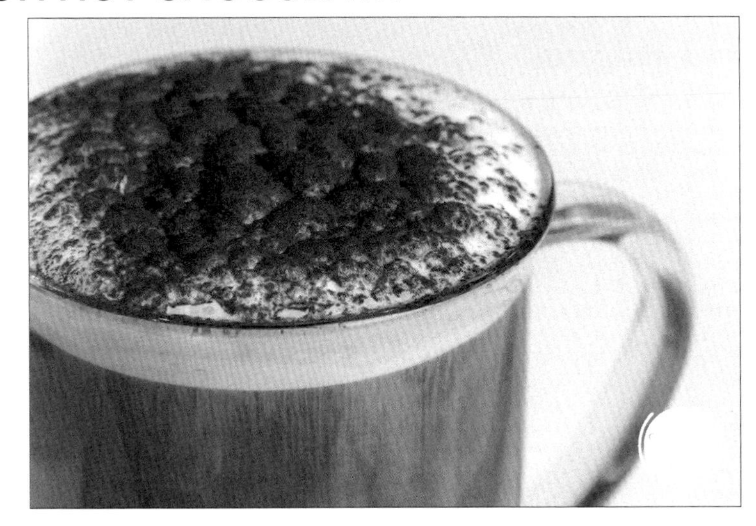

WHAT YOU NEED

- 1 cup / 8 fl oz almond milk
- ½ cup / 4 fl oz water
- ¼ cup / 2 fl oz heavy cream
- ½ TBSP unsweetened cocoa powder
- 1 tsp ground cinnamon
- 2 tsp vanilla extract
- 2 TBSP xylitol or erythritol
- small pinch of sea salt
- ½ oz / 15 g 100% unsweetened chocolate, chopped

WHAT YOU DO

1. Place the almond milk, water, cream, cocoa powder, cinnamon, vanilla extract, xylitol or erythritol, and sea salt in a pan over medium heat, whisk well and heat until it starts to steam.
2. Turn off the heat and add the chopped chocolate, stirring until completely melted and mixed through.
3. While it is still in the pan, whisk the hot chocolate using a handheld frother or immersion blender for several minutes until it is completely smooth and frothy.

NOTES

- The cinnamon will give this a slightly grainy feel as it does not fully dissolve in hot liquid. You could replace the ground cinnamon with 1 tsp of cinnamon extract if the graininess bothers you.

BAKED CHEESE & BACON BREAKFAST PIE

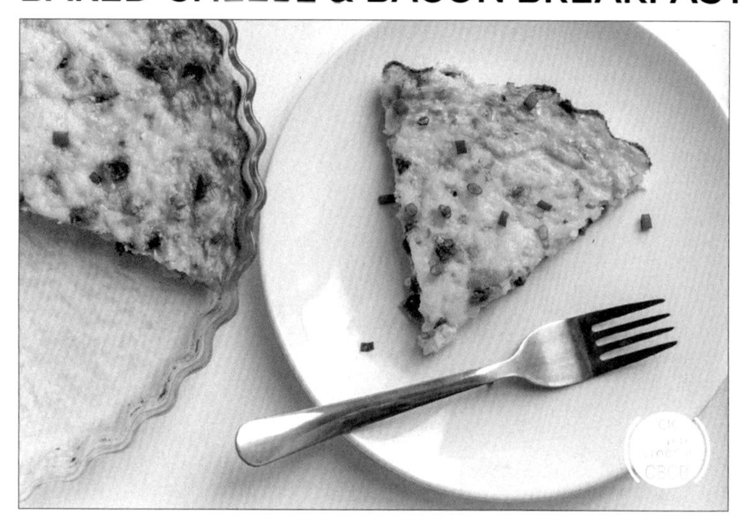

Servings:
2
Category:
Meal 1
Prep time:
10 minutes
Cook time:
50 - 60 minutes
Total time:
1 hour 10 minutes
CertifiedKetogenic.com **Rating:**
Certified Ketogenic

WHAT YOU NEED

3 eggs

2 TBSP / 1 fl oz heavy cream

2 TBSP / 1 fl oz water

2 oz / 55 g bacon, cooked and roughly chopped or crumbled

4 oz / 110 g riced cauliflower

2 oz / 55 g mozzarella, grated

2 oz / 55 g full fat cottage cheese

1 tsp dried oregano

2 scallions (green / spring onions)

ground black pepper

½ oz / 15 g Cheddar cheese, grated

WHAT YOU DO

1. Spray a baking dish with coconut oil.
2. In a large bowl whisk the eggs, cream, and water very well and then stir in the chopped bacon, cauliflower, grated mozzarella, cottage cheese, dried oregano, onions and pepper and mix well until completely combined.
3. Pour mixture into greased baking dish. Sprinkle with grated Cheddar.
4. Bake at 325°F for 50 to 60 minutes, until golden brown.

NOTES

- You can make this the night before, cover and keep in the 'fridge and bake in the morning.
- Extra servings can be frozen. Cut into individual portions before putting in the freezer. To thaw, defrost overnight in the fridge and then reheat gently in the toaster oven or microwave.

HAM, LEEK & FETA EGG CUPS

Servings:
1
Category:
Meal 1
Prep time:
15 minutes
Cook time:
30 minutes
Total time:
45 minutes
CertifiedKetogenic.com **Rating:**
Certified Ketogenic

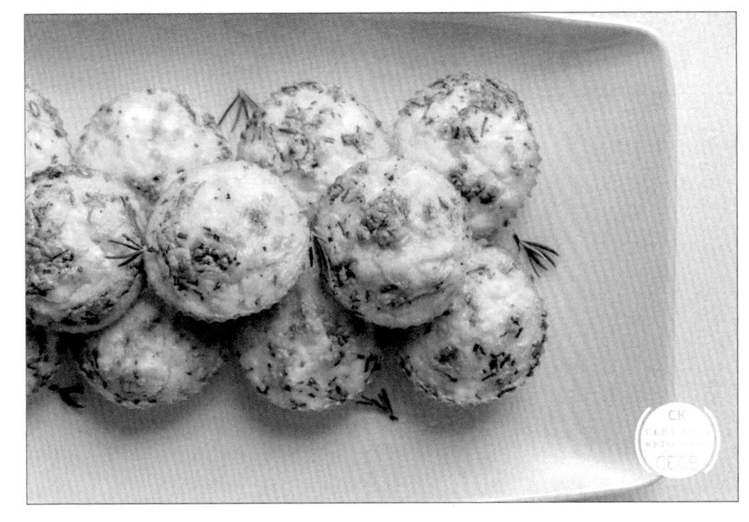

WHAT YOU NEED

1 TBSP avocado oil

6 oz / 170g leeks, finely sliced

6 oz / 170 g ham, sliced or chopped

4 oz / 110 g feta cheese, cut into small cubes

9 eggs

2 TBSP heavy cream

1 TBSP fresh rosemary, finely chopped

ground black pepper

WHAT YOU DO

1. Spray 12 silicone muffin cups or a muffin tin with avocado oil.
2. Heat the avocado oil in a pan and sauté the leeks and ham together over medium heat until the leeks are soft.
3. Divide the leek and ham mixture evenly between the 12 muffin cups.
4. Divide the feta evenly between the 12 muffin cups.
5. In a large jug whisk the eggs, cream, fresh rosemary, and pepper until completely mixed.
6. Carefully pour the egg mixture equally into the muffin cups over the leeks, ham and feta.
7. Bake in the center of the oven at 375°F for 30 minutes until well-risen and golden brown.
8. Can be eaten hot or cold. Store in an airtight container in the 'fridge.

NOTES

- Extra servings can be frozen. To thaw, defrost overnight in the fridge and then reheat gently in the toaster oven or microwave.

EGG & BACON SALAD

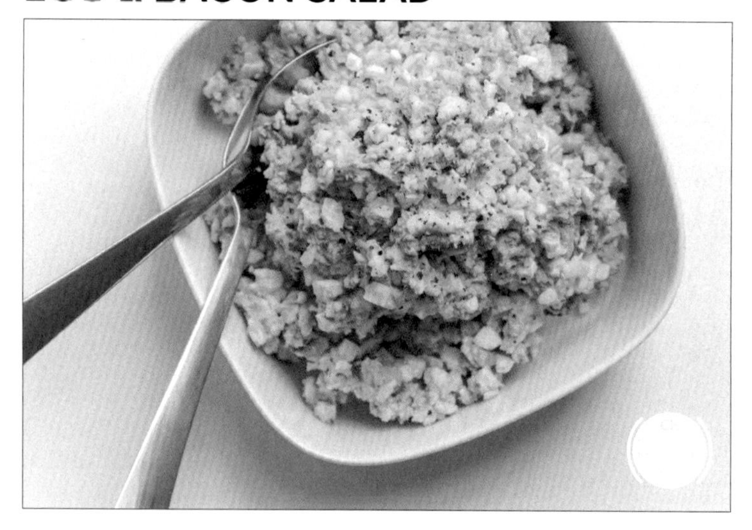

Servings:
2
Category:
Meal 1
Prep time:
10 minutes
Cook time:
15 minutes
Total time:
25 minutes
CertifiedKetogenic.com **Rating:**
Certified Ketogenic

WHAT YOU NEED

6 eggs
4 oz / 110 g bacon
1 TBSP tomato paste
1 oz / 30 g butter, softened
2 TBSP heavy cream
sea salt
ground black pepper
½ tsp lemon juice

WHAT YOU DO

1. Cook the bacon and chop or crumble depending on how crispy you cooked it.
2. Meanwhile, hard-boil the eggs, cool, and peel.
3. Place the eggs in a large bowl and chop finely using a knife. It's easier to contain the eggs if you do the chopping in a bowl.
4. Add the chopped or crumbled bacon, tomato paste, softened butter, cream, sea salt, pepper and lemon juice and mix very well until completely combined.
5. Store in an airtight container in the 'fridge.

PORK LOVER'S SCRAMBLE

Servings:
1
Category:
Meal 1
Prep time:
5 minutes
Cook time:
10 minutes
Total time:
15 minutes
CertifiedKetogenic.com **Rating:**
Certified Ketogenic

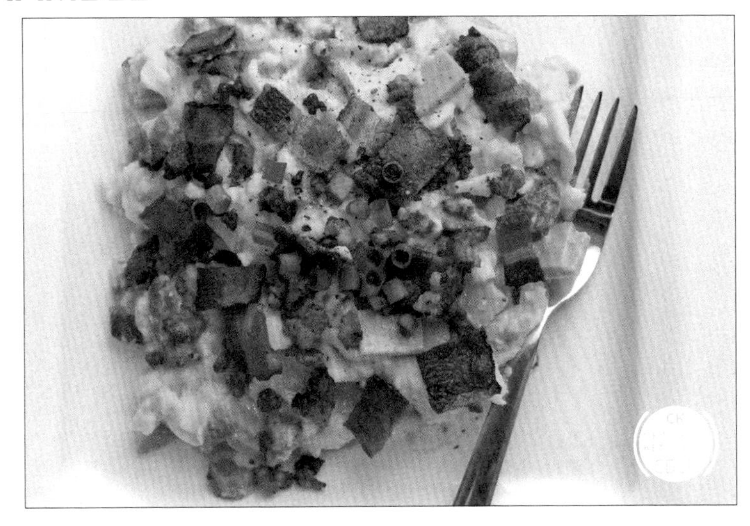

WHAT YOU NEED

2 oz / 55 g ground pork (sausage meat)

1 oz / 30 g ham, chopped

1 ½ oz / 42 g bacon, chopped

3 eggs

1 TBSP heavy cream

sea salt

ground black pepper

WHAT YOU DO

1. In a frying pan, sauté the pork, ham, and bacon until cooked through and nicely browned. Remove from pan and reserve. Return the pan to the heat.
2. Whisk the eggs, cream, sea salt and pepper together well in a jug.
3. Pour the whisked egg mixture into the pan you used to sauté the meats and stir constantly over a medium heat until the eggs are almost cooked to the firmness that you like.
4. Add the meats to the eggs and stir well.
5. Remove from the heat when the eggs are cooked but still glossy and moist.
6. Serve immediately.

SALMON AVOCADO OMELET

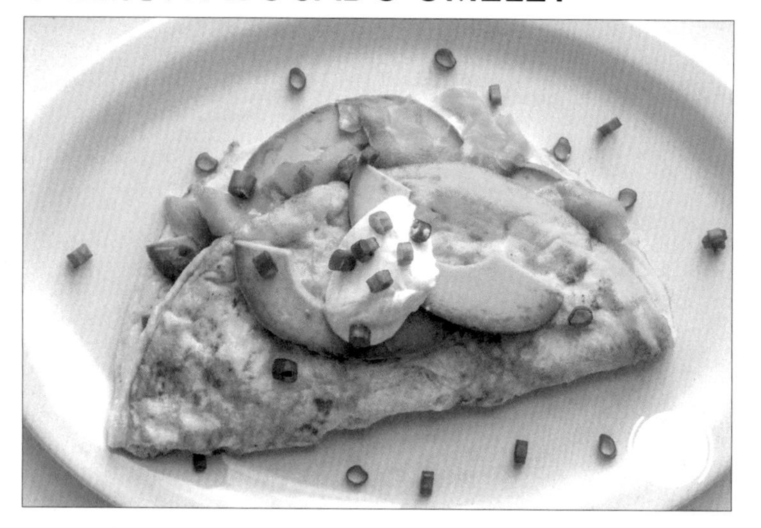

Servings:
1
Category:
Meal 1
Prep time:
5 minutes
Cook time:
3 minutes
Total time:
8 minutes
CertifiedKetogenic.com **Rating:**
Certified Ketogenic

WHAT YOU NEED

2 TBSP lemon juice

½ avocado

3 eggs

sea salt

ground black pepper

1 oz / 30 g cream cheese, chopped into small pieces

1 ½ oz / 42 g smoked salmon (lox), very finely sliced

1 scallion (green or spring onion) finely sliced

WHAT YOU DO

1. Put the lemon juice in a small bowl. Cut the avocado in half, remove the stone, peel, slice and then toss the avocado slices in the lemon juice until completely coated.
2. Put a frying pan over high heat for a minute and also turn on the broiler (grill). Whisk the eggs, sea salt and pepper well in a small jug. Add the pieces of cream cheese and stir well.
3. Pour the egg mixture into the hot pan and cook without stirring for 30 seconds until the outer 1/8 inch of the edge is firm. The middle will still appear to be completely fluid.
4. Remove pan from the heat and put under the hot broiler (grill) until the top of the omelet is just set (about 45 seconds).
5. Remove from under the broiler (grill), shake the pan to free the omelet, and place pan back on the stove.
6. Add the salmon and avocado slices to one half of the omelet, then slide the omelet on a plate (filled side first) and flip the empty side of the omelet over the avocado and salmon. Sprinkle with onion and serve immediately.

MUSHROOM & PANCETTA FRITTATA

Servings:
2
Category:
Meal 1
Prep time:
5 minutes
Cook time:
10 minutes
Total time:
15 minutes
CertifiedKetogenic.com **Rating:**
Certified Ketogenic

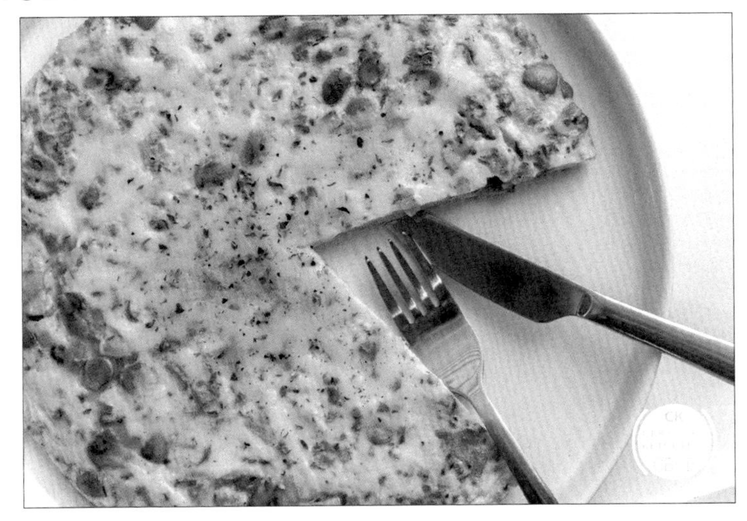

WHAT YOU NEED

4 oz / 110 g mushrooms, chopped

4 oz / 110 g pancetta, chopped

8 eggs

2 TBSP heavy cream

6 TBSP water

sea salt

ground black pepper

1 tsp dried oregano

1 oz / 30 g Cheddar cheese, grated

WHAT YOU DO

1. Sauté the chopped mushrooms and pancetta over a medium heat until the mushrooms are just softened.
2. Turn the broiler (grill) on to heat.
3. Meanwhile, whisk the eggs, cream, water, sea salt and pepper, and oregano in a jug until completely mixed.
4. Pour the egg mixture into the pan over the mushrooms and pancetta and stir for 30 seconds while the eggs start to cook.
5. After 30 seconds, stop stirring and leave to cook for a further 2 minutes.
6. Remove from the heat and place under the broiler (grill) until the top is set and just starting to brown.
7. Remove from under the broiler (grill), sprinkle top with grated Cheddar and slide onto a large plate or serving dish. Slice to serve.

NOTES

- Extra servings can be frozen. Cut into individual portions before putting in the freezer. Defrost overnight in the fridge, then reheat gently in the toaster oven or microwave.

PECAN NUTMEG "OATMEAL"

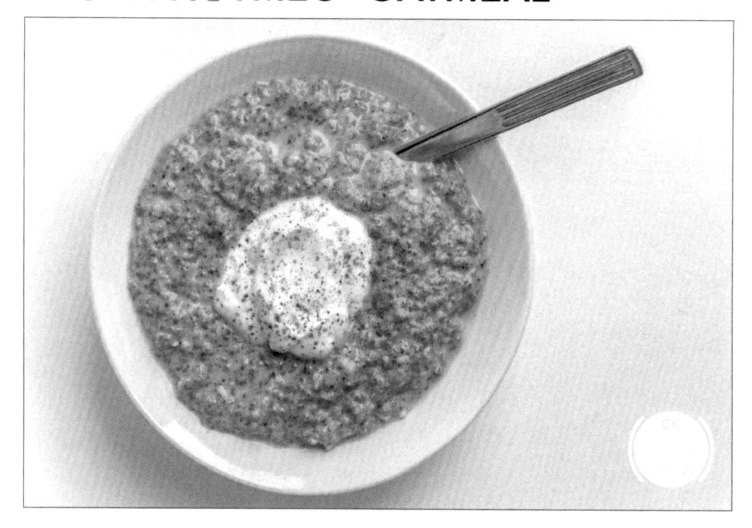

Servings:
2
Category:
Meal 1
Prep time:
5 minutes
Cook time:
2 minutes
Total time:
7 minutes
CertifiedKetogenic.com **Rating:**
Certified Ketogenic

WHAT YOU NEED

4 TBSP sunflower seeds

2 TBSP unsweetened, shredded coconut

2 TBSP chia seeds

6 TBSP finely chopped toasted pecans

1 tsp ground nutmeg

1 oz / 30 g egg white powder

¾ cup / 6 fl oz boiling water

1 tsp vanilla extract

2 tsp xylitol or erythritol (or more to taste)

WHAT YOU DO

1. Place sunflower seeds, shredded coconut, and chia seeds in a coffee grinder or food processor and grind until fine. (If you use a high-powered blender, be careful you don't end up with a paste!)
2. Pour ground seed mix into a bowl, add the finely chopped toasted pecans, ground nutmeg and protein powder and stir well until completely blended.
3. Add boiling water and stir well. Leave to sit for one minute to thicken. Stir and add more boiling water if you prefer a runnier "oatmeal".
4. Add the vanilla extract and either xylitol or erythritol to sweeten to taste, and serve with a dollop of sour cream or Greek yogurt if you feel so moved. It's delicious with sour cream.

NOTES

- For one serving, use half the mix and add ⅜ cup / 3 fl oz boiling water.

NO MORE DEATH BY CHOCOLATE FRAPPE

Servings:
1
Category:
Meal 1
Prep time:
5 minutes
Cook time:
0 minutes
Total time:
5 minutes
CertifiedKetogenic.com **Rating:**
Certified Ketogenic

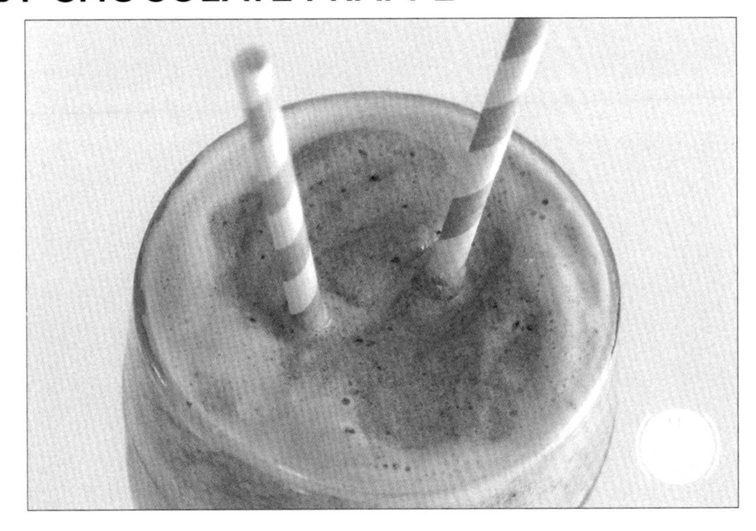

WHAT YOU NEED

1 cup ice cubes

1 oz / 30 g 100% unsweetened chocolate, chopped

3 TBSP unsweetened cocoa powder

4 TBSP xylitol or erythritol (or to taste)

2 pinches of sea salt

½ cup / 4 fl oz unsweetened almond milk

½ cup / 4 fl oz **cold** strong coffee

¼ tsp guar gum (optional, but highly recommended – improves texture)

WHAT YOU DO

1. Place ingredients – except guar gum – in a blender and blend until ice is smooth.
2. Tap the guar gum through the hole in the lid while blender is running and blend for 5 seconds.

NOTES

- To save time, you can use store-bought cold brew coffee instead of brewing coffee and then chilling it before use. Check the ingredients to make sure it only has coffee in.

CREAMY LEMON COCONUT CEREAL

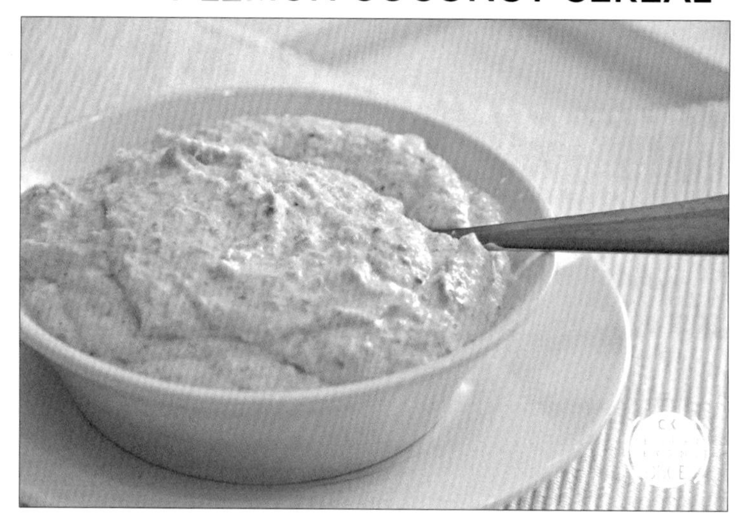

Servings:
2
Category:
Meal 1
Prep time:
5 minutes
Cook time:
0 minutes
Total time:
5 minutes
CertifiedKetogenic.com **Rating:**
Certified Ketogenic

WHAT YOU NEED

1 TBSP chia seeds

2 TBSP sunflower seeds

4 TBSP unsweetened shredded coconut

1 oz / 28 g egg white powder

1 TBSP xylitol or erythritol (add more to taste)

1/2 TBSP lemon zest (1/2 lemon)

2 tsp lemon juice

1 cup / 8 fl oz plain, unsweetened full-fat Greek yogurt

¼ cup / 2 fl oz unsweetened almond milk

WHAT YOU DO

1. Grind chia, sunflower seeds and coconut until very fine in a coffee grinder or high-speed blender (be careful you don't end up with sunflower butter!).
2. In a bowl, add ground seed mix, egg white powder, xylitol or erythritol, and mix well.
3. Add the lemon zest, lemon juice, yogurt, and almond milk. Stir thoroughly until completely mixed.

NOTES

- Store extra in a covered container in the fridge.

COCONUT LIME LASSI

Servings:
1
Category:
Meal 1
Prep time:
3 minutes
Cook time:
0 minutes
Total time:
3 minutes
CertifiedKetogenic.com **Rating:**
Certified Ketogenic

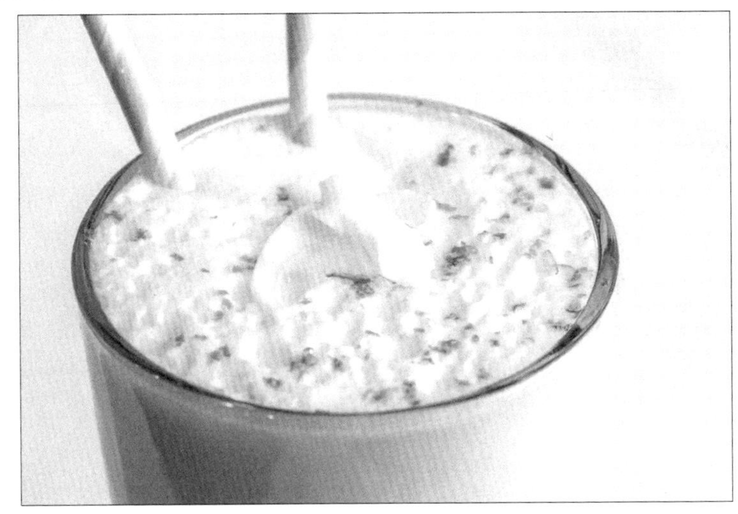

WHAT YOU NEED

½ cup / 4 fl oz plain, unsweetened full-fat Greek yogurt

½ cup / 4 fl oz canned unsweetened full-fat thick coconut milk

1 cup / 8 fl oz cold water

1 TBSP (or to taste) xylitol or erythritol

2 tsp lime juice

WHAT YOU DO

1. Place all the ingredients into a blender and blend for 5 seconds.
2. Pour into a glass and serve

MEAL 2 SELECTIONS

Just Don't Call It a Snack

Meal 2 is totally, completely, 100% optional. After switching to keto from a SAD lifestyle, you may feel very hungry mid-day and need some additional fuel. You may struggle with changing your routine and feel "like you should eat." In these moments, this list will get you through.

As your body becomes fat-adapted, however, don't be surprised if Meal 2 fades into distant memory. Intermittent fasting is built into a keto lifestyle, and often we go about our day on nothing but a cup of coffee, only to realize it's late evening and we are hungry for our **first** meal of the day!

If you do find yourself only eating one or two meals a day, there's nothing to worry about as long as you're getting enough food to keep your metabolism functioning. If you are a very busy person, you may also prefer to replace a meal with a few items on this list for convenience's sake.

Pick any combination from this list to satiety:

- Hard-boiled eggs
- Cheese (slices or string)
- Plain, unsweetened Greek yogurt
- Jerky
- Nuts (macadamia, pili, or hazelnut)
- An avocado
- Small can of sardines or salmon
- Salami slices
- Sliced deli meats
- Pork rinds
- Cream cheese-filled celery sticks
- Leftovers from a recipe in this book

Note on ingredients: If you purchase any of these items pre-packaged, be sure to check the labels for sugar, fillers, and other unnecessary and/or suspect ingredients. They should contain only the ingredients you would use if you made them yourself. Jerky is a particularly tough one to find with keto-friendly ingredients, so start at the natural health food stores.

Lifestyle tip: A very common question from folks new to keto is, "What should I eat at the movie theater?" This of course assumes you are actually **hungry** when you're at the theater. Always be careful to avoid mindless eating! With a couple obvious, more fragrant, exceptions (to avoid your theater-going neighbors coming at you with pitchforks), this Meal 2 list is a great place to look for your new favorite theater food. Smuggle it in using someone's purse if your theater forbids outside food but won't provide healthy options. There is also the Vanilla Hazelnut Granola from page 111 which will make everyone jealous!

ONE-PAN DINNERS

While it is possible to spend all day slaving over a hot oven to craft a delectable spread of ketogenic food, when you're trying to start out, there's no point in making things more complicated than they have to be. On the following pages, you'll find recipes for mouth-watering dishes which combine ingredients and textures in satisfying ways, without needing to involve every burner on the stove, every rack of the oven, and every appliance in the cabinet.

These recipes are great for making ahead, and they store or freeze well.

PRAWNS WITH LEEKS & LEMON PEPPER

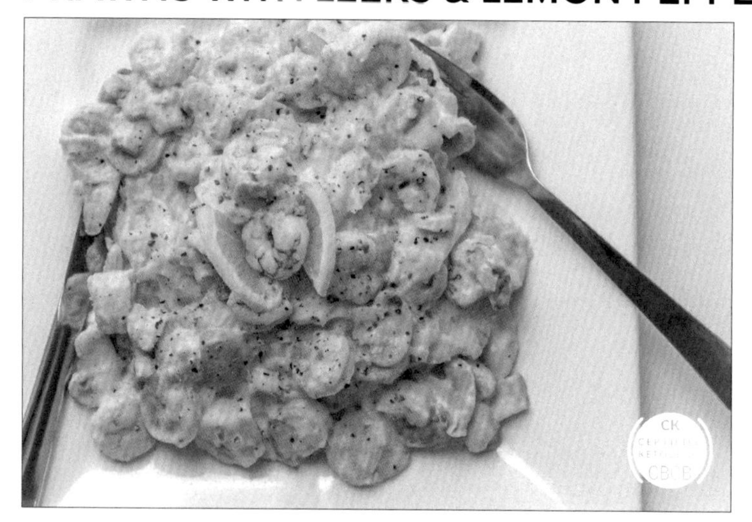

Servings:
2
Category:
One Pan Meal
Prep time:
5 minutes
Cook time:
10 minutes
Total time:
15 minutes
CertifiedKetogenic.com **Rating:**
Certified Ketogenic

WHAT YOU NEED

1 TBSP avocado oil

6 oz / 170 g leeks, sliced

4 oz / 110 g mushrooms, sliced

12 oz / 335 g prawns (shrimp), pre-cooked, de-veined, tail-off

⅓ cup / 3 fl oz plain, unsweetened full-fat Greek yogurt (Non-fat will not work!)

1 TBSP lemon juice

lemon pepper

WHAT YOU DO

1. Heat the avocado oil in a large skillet and sauté the leeks gently over a medium heat, stirring often, for about 5 minutes until the leeks are tender.
2. Add the sliced mushrooms to the skillet and cook for 1 minute.
3. Add the prawns and heat through.
4. Add the Greek yogurt to the skillet and toss the prawn mixture until it is evenly coated in yogurt.
5. Stir in the lemon juice.
6. Season liberally with fresh ground lemon pepper and spoon onto plates.

WARM TURKEY & ALMOND SLAW

Servings:
2
Category:
One Pan Meal
Prep time:
5 minutes
Cook time:
5 minutes
Total time:
10 minutes
CertifiedKetogenic.com **Rating:**
Certified Ketogenic

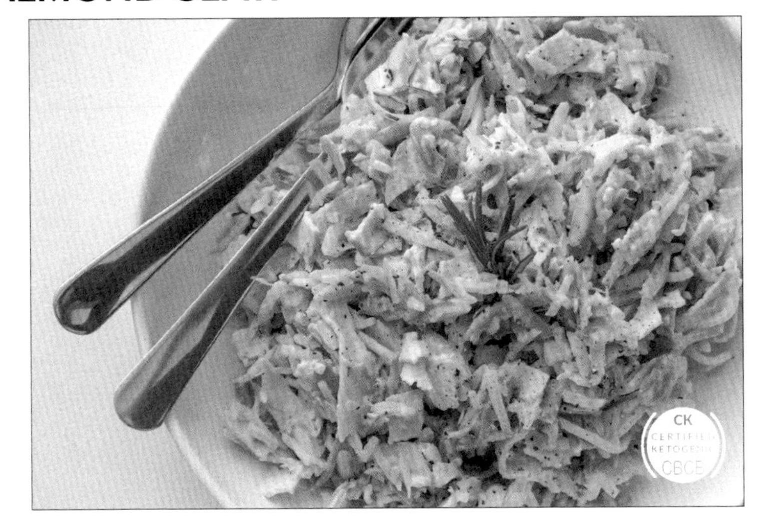

WHAT YOU NEED

1 TBSP avocado oil

6 oz / 170g broccoli slaw

2 oz / 55g slivered (not flaked) toasted almonds

7 oz / 195g packet smoked deli turkey, sliced into thin strips

2 tsp fresh rosemary

¼ cup / 2 fl oz plain, unsweetened full-fat Greek yogurt (Non-fat will not work!)

1 TBSP white wine vinegar

1 TBSP heavy cream

ground black pepper

sea salt

WHAT YOU DO

1. Heat the avocado oil in a skillet over high heat.
2. Add the broccoli slaw and the almonds and stir-fry for 2 minutes, stirring constantly.
3. Reduce the heat to medium.
4. Add the strips of turkey, stir and cook for 1 minute.
5. Add the fresh rosemary, yogurt, white wine vinegar, cream, sea salt, and pepper and stir gently until completely combined.

NOTES

- Carrots contain sugars and are not normally part of a ketogenic diet. If you cannot get broccoli slaw without a tiny amount of carrots included, you can fish out the few bits of carrot either before you cook, or as you eat.

CREAMY CHICKEN & CABBAGE CASSEROLE

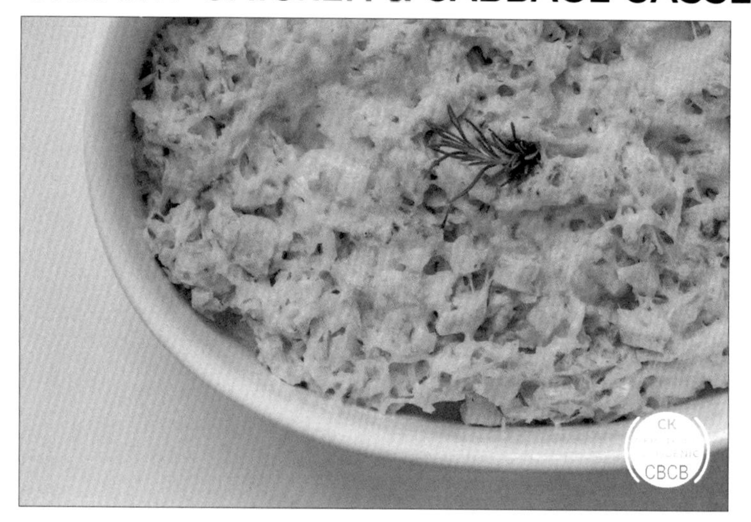

Servings:
2
Category:
One Pan Meal
Prep time:
5 minutes
Cook time:
15 minutes
Total time:
20 minutes
CertifiedKetogenic.com **Rating:**
Certified Ketogenic

WHAT YOU NEED

1 TBSP avocado oil

8 oz / 225 g trimmed leeks, very finely sliced

Sea salt and ground pepper to taste

10 oz / 280 g cabbage, very finely shredded

1 lb / 450 g cooked chicken, cut into small pieces

1 TBSP fresh rosemary, finely chopped

¼ cup / 2 fl oz heavy cream

2 oz / 55 g cream cheese

1 oz / 30 g Cheddar cheese, grated

WHAT YOU DO

1. Heat the avocado oil in a large pan over a medium heat, add the leeks, sea salt and pepper and sauté for 5 minutes.
2. Add the shredded cabbage, stir well, and sauté for a further 5 minutes.
3. Add the cooked chicken pieces, fresh rosemary, cream, and cream cheese to the pan and stir well until the cream cheese has completely melted and coats the chicken and veggies.
4. Spoon the mix into a casserole dish, cover with the grated cheese and broil (grill) until golden brown.

CHICKEN & AVOCADO SALAD

Servings:
2
Category:
One Pan Meal
Prep time:
15 minutes
Cook time:
0 minutes
Total time:
15 minutes
CertifiedKetogenic.com **Rating:**
Certified Ketogenic

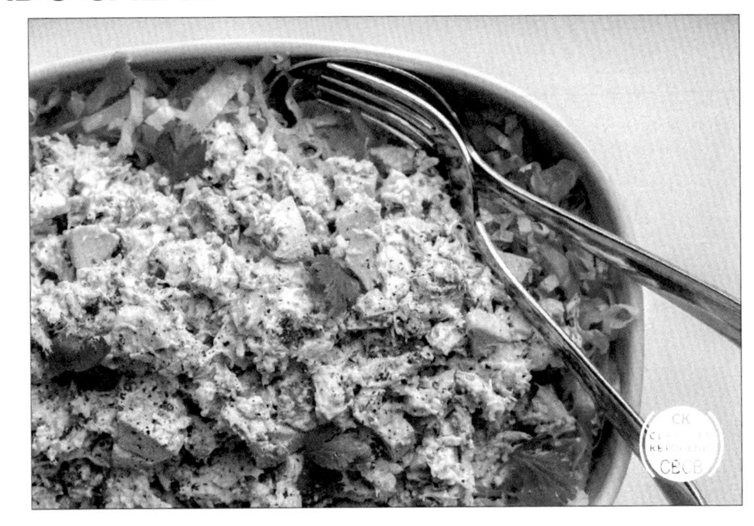

WHAT YOU NEED

- 2 TBSP / 1 fl oz water
- ¼ cup / 2 fl oz sour cream
- 2 TBSP / 1 fl oz heavy cream
- 1 TBSP fresh cilantro, finely chopped
- ¼ tsp sea salt
- 2 scallions (green / spring onions)
- 1 TBSP lime juice
- 8 oz / 225 g cooked chicken, chopped into pieces
- 4 oz / 110 g cooked bacon, chopped into pieces
- 1 avocado, cut lengthwise, stone removed, peeled, and cut into pieces.
- romaine lettuce, shredded

WHAT YOU DO

1. In a large bowl combine the water, sour cream, cream, cilantro, sea salt and onions and mix well.
2. Add the lime juice, cooked chicken, cooked bacon, and avocado and stir gently until everything is completely coated in cream mixture.
3. Place the shredded lettuce on a plate and spoon the chicken avocado mixture on top.

NOTES

- Keep any leftover chicken salad in a covered container in the fridge.

DOUBLE PORK FRIED “RICE”

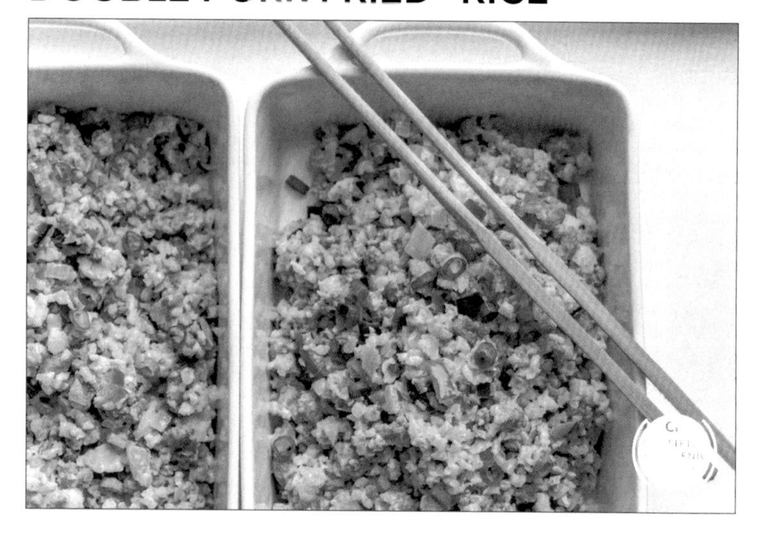

Servings:
2
Category:
One Pan Meal
Prep time:
10 minutes
Cook time:
30 minutes
Total time:
40 minutes
CertifiedKetogenic.com **Rating:**
Certified Ketogenic

WHAT YOU NEED

8 oz / 225 g ground pork (sausage meat)

3 oz / 85 g bacon, chopped

2 ½ oz / 70 g onions, finely chopped

4 oz / 110 g riced cauliflower

1 ½ oz / 42 g red pepper, chopped

2 eggs, whisked

1 oz / 30 g cream cheese

2 TBSP / 1 fl oz heavy cream

WHAT YOU DO

1. Cook the sausage in a pan over medium heat, breaking up the meat into very small pieces with a spatula as it cooks. Once it is browned, remove meat from the pan and reserve, leaving the fat in the pan.
2. Cook the chopped bacon and onions in the fat in the pan for 5 minutes.
3. Add the riced cauliflower and red pepper and cook for a further 10 minutes, stirring frequently.
4. Meanwhile, pour the eggs into in a separate sauté pan and leave them to cook for 30 seconds, then move the eggs around. Let cook, stirring occasionally, for another minute until the eggs are dry. Remove from the heat and “chop” the eggs into small pieces with a spatula while they are still in the pan.
5. Add the pork back into the pan with the vegetables and stir well. Turn the heat to low.
6. Stir the cream cheese, cream, and cooked eggs into the sausage mixture until the cream cheese is completely melted and everything is mixed in.

MONTANA HASH

Servings:
2
Category:
One Pan Meal
Prep time:
10 minutes
Cook time:
30 minutes
Total time:
40 minutes
CertifiedKetogenic.com **Rating:**
Certified Ketogenic

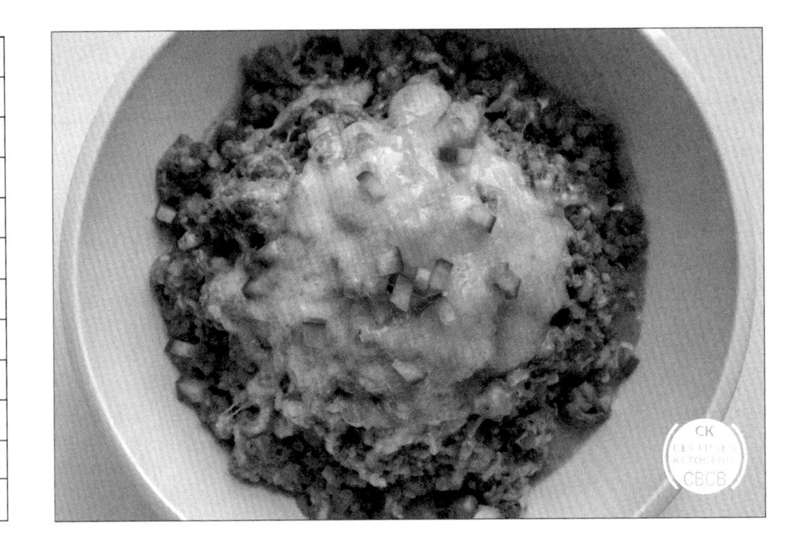

WHAT YOU NEED

1 TBSP avocado oil

2 cloves fresh garlic, crushed

1 ¾ oz / 50 g onion, finely chopped

1 ½ oz / 42 g green pepper, finely chopped

8 oz / 225 g ground beef (minced beef)

5 oz / 140 g riced cauliflower

1 tsp Dijon mustard

1 tsp sea salt

ground black pepper

1 TBSP tomato paste

½ cup / 4 fl oz beef stock

3 TBSP / 1 ½ fl oz heavy cream

1 oz / 30 g Cheddar cheese, grated

WHAT YOU DO

1. Heat the avocado oil over medium heat, add the crushed garlic, chopped onion and green pepper and sauté for 5 minutes until softened.
2. Add the ground beef and sauté for a further 5 minutes until it is no longer pink, breaking up the meat into very small pieces with a spatula as it cooks.
3. Add the riced cauliflower, mustard, salt, pepper, tomato paste, beef stock, and cream, bring to a boil, reduce heat and simmer for 20 minutes.
4. Sprinkle grated cheese on top and serve.

CREAMY CAJUN SAUSAGE SKILLET

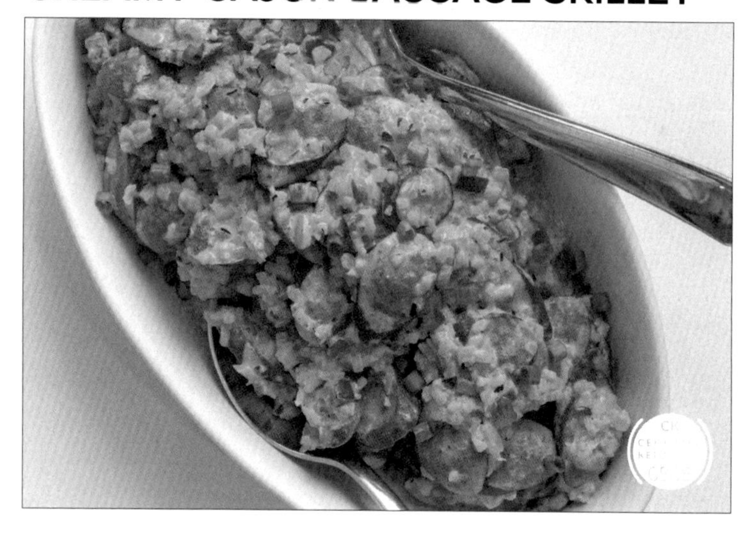

Servings:
2
Category:
One Pan Meal
Prep time:
10 minutes
Cook time:
30 minutes
Total time:
40 minutes
CertifiedKetogenic.com **Rating:**
Certified Ketogenic

WHAT YOU NEED

1 TBSP avocado oil

1 oz / 30 g onion, finely chopped

1 oz / 30 g red pepper, finely chopped

4 oz / 110 g riced cauliflower

¼ cup / 2 fl oz chicken stock

½ tsp salt

¼ tsp cayenne pepper

½ tsp smoked paprika

¼ tsp ground black pepper

¼ tsp onion powder

¼ tsp dried oregano

¼ tsp dried thyme

8 oz / 225 g cooked sausage, sliced diagonally in ¼" slices

2 oz / 55 g cream cheese

WHAT YOU DO

1. Heat the avocado oil in a pan over medium heat and sauté the onions for 5 minutes. Add the red pepper, riced cauliflower, chicken stock, salt and all the spices and herbs.
2. Bring to the boil, then reduce heat and simmer for 20 minutes.
3. Add the sliced cooked sausage and mix well.
4. Add the cream cheese and stir until completely melted and everything is coated in melted cheese.

PROTEINS

A simple way to add variety into any nutritional lifestyle is to mix and match proteins and side dishes. In Chapter 10, you'll find instructions to cook common proteins which highlight their natural flavor and textures.

In Chapter 11, you'll find a bevy of side dish recipes to pair with these proteins for a complete keto profile on a plate.

These serve as alternative dinners to the One Pan Meal recipes of the previous chapter. They are sized for one serving to provide variety, but if you buy a tray of multiple pieces, wrap the extras well and freeze them to use again.

PORK CHOPS

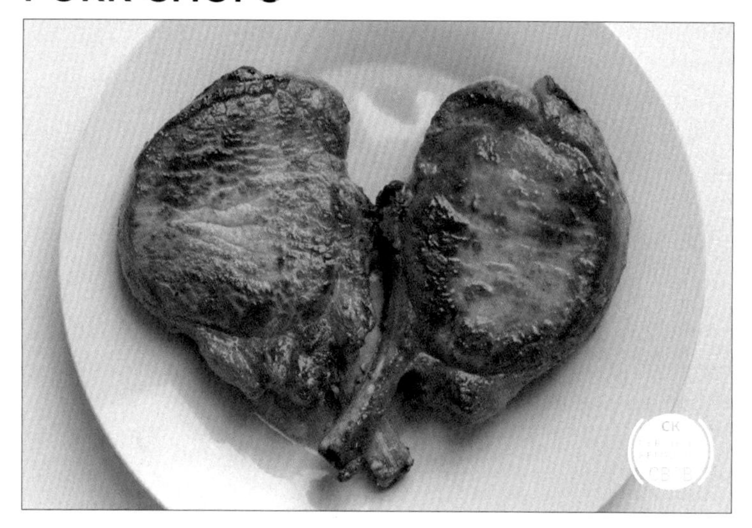

Servings:
1
Category:
Protein
Prep time:
0 minutes
Cook time:
10 minutes
Total time:
10 minutes
CertifiedKetogenic.com **Rating:**
Certified Ketogenic

WHAT YOU NEED

1 pork chop

WHAT YOU DO

1. Remove the skillet or pan from the cupboard and the pork chop from the 'fridge.
2. Put the **cold** pork chop (no oil or fat needed) in the **cold** skillet and place the **cold** skillet on the **cold** stove.
3. Turn the heat on medium.
4. Cook for 3 minutes on each side, searing with a spatula after flipping. **Do not touch.** Walk away if you have to.
5. Cook for 2 minutes on each side, searing with a spatula after flipping. **Do not touch between flips.** Walk away if you have to.
6. Cook for 1 minute on each side, searing with a spatula after flipping. **Do not touch between flips.** You're almost done!
7. Slide onto your plate and watch in awe as a few minutes later the juices start to ooze out the sides.
8. Eat the juiciest pork chop you've ever had in your life.

NOTES

- Cooking time will vary dependent on thickness of your chop and whether it has a bone in. The chop is done when it is perfectly browned on both sides.

STEAK

Servings:
2
Category:
Protein
Prep time:
5 minutes
Cook time:
5-10 minutes
Total time:
10-15 minutes
CertifiedKetogenic.com **Rating:**
Certified Ketogenic

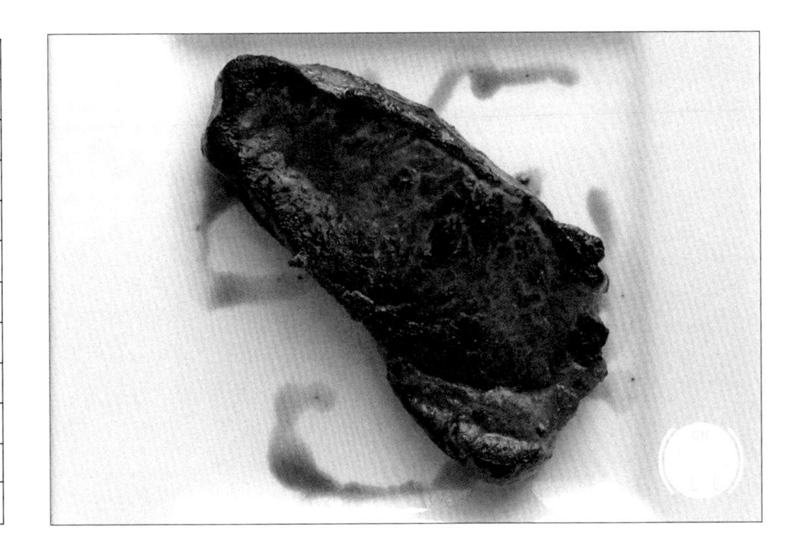

WHAT YOU NEED

1 steak
2 TBSP avocado oil
sea salt
ground black pepper

WHAT YOU DO

1. If you know how to grill a steak well, go right ahead. If you're not a confident griller and / or you don't have a grill, here's how to cook a steak in your oven.
2. Pre-heat oven to 400°F.
3. Place avocado oil in a skillet (with an oven-proof handle) and heat on high until very hot.
4. When the oil starts to steam, season the steak on each side with sea salt and ground black pepper and carefully lower steak into pan and cook for 1 minute on each side.
5. Place the skillet in the oven and close the door.
6. Cook for 3 to 7 more minutes depending how you like your steak:
   - Rare: 3 minutes
   - Medium rare: 5 minutes
   - Medium: 7 minutes
7. Carefully remove pan from over using oven mitts – remember the handle is now 400°F!!
8. Let the steak rest for 2 minutes before serving.

SALMON

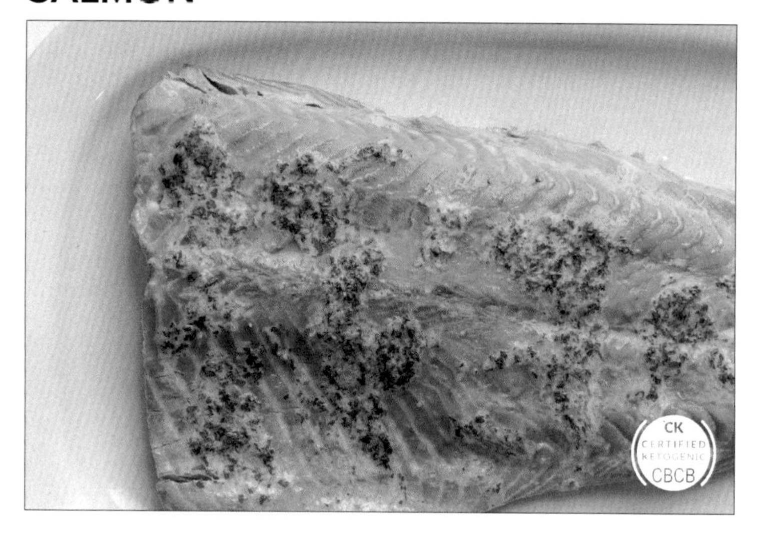

Servings:
1
Category:
Protein
Prep time:
5 minutes
Cook time:
12 minutes
Total time:
17 minutes
CertifiedKetogenic.com **Rating:**
Certified Ketogenic

WHAT YOU NEED

1 salmon fillet

2 TBSP butter

WHAT YOU DO

1. Put butter on a rimmed cookie sheet or pan and place in the center of the oven at 475°F for one minute just until the butter melts. Carefully remove the sheet from the oven. Don't forget the oven gloves.
2. Season the top of your salmon fillet evenly with sea salt and ground black pepper. Using a spatula, carefully slide the salmon fillet – skin side down – into the melted butter and then return the sheet to the oven.
3. Roast the salmon until just cooked – about 8 to 12 minutes depending on how thick your fillet is. The salmon will flake easily when cooked.

LAMB CHOPS

Servings:
1
Category:
Protein
Prep time:
0 minutes
Cook time:
12 minutes
Total time:
12 minutes
CertifiedKetogenic.com **Rating:**
Certified Ketogenic

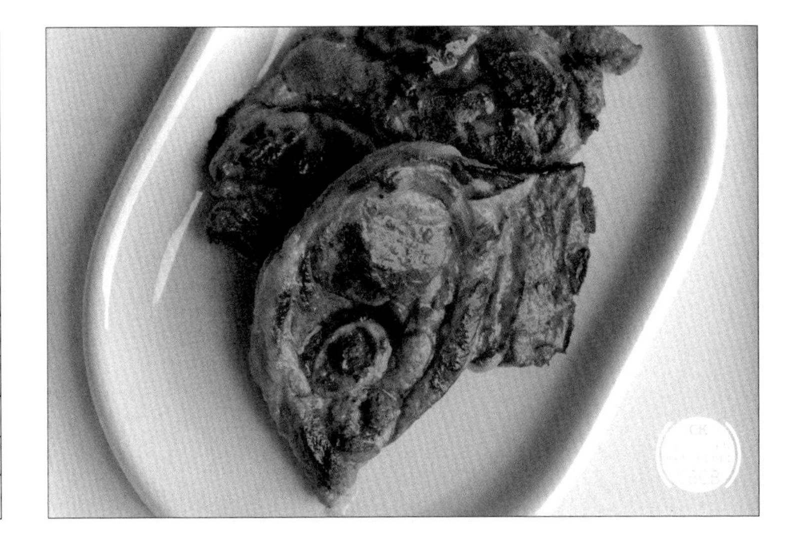

WHAT YOU NEED

1 lamb chop

WHAT YOU DO

1. Heat pan over a medium heat.
2. Add lamb chop and cook for one minute on each side.
3. Reduce heat to medium low and cook chop for 5 minutes or until browned on the bottom.
4. Turn the chop over and cook for a further 5 minutes until that side is also browned.

NOTES

- Cooking time will vary dependent on thickness of the chop and whether it has a bone in. They are done when they are perfectly browned on both sides.

PORK SHOULDER

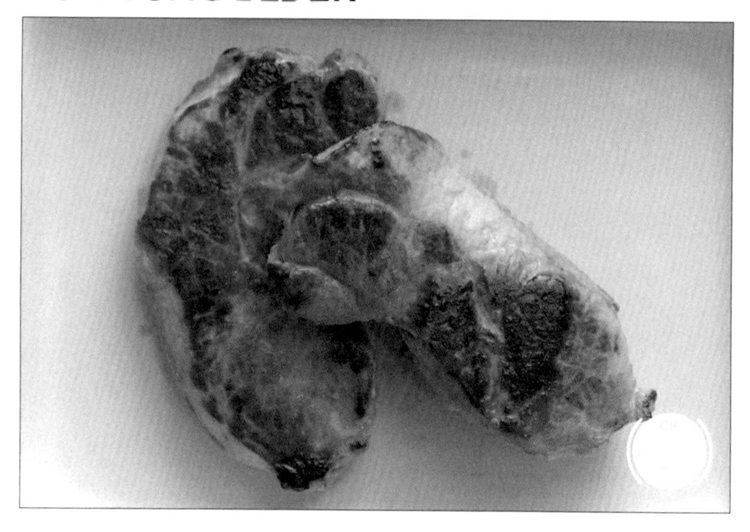

Servings:
1
Category:
Protein
Prep time:
0 minutes
Cook time:
10 minutes
Total time:
10 minutes
CertifiedKetogenic.com **Rating:**
Certified Ketogenic

WHAT YOU NEED

1 pork shoulder chop

WHAT YOU DO

1. Remove the skillet or pan from the cupboard and the pork shoulder chop from the 'fridge.
2. Put the **cold** pork chop (no oil or fat needed) in the **cold** skillet and place the **cold** skillet on the **cold** stove.
3. Turn the heat on medium.
4. Cook for 3 minutes on each side, searing with a spatula after flipping. Do not touch. Walk away if you have to.
5. Cook for 2 minutes on each side, searing with a spatula after flipping. Do not touch between flips. Walk away if you have to.
6. Cook for 1 minute on each side, searing with a spatula after flipping. Do not touch between flips. You're almost done!
7. Slide onto your plate and watch in awe as a few minutes later the juices start to ooze out the sides.
8. Eat the juiciest pork chop you've ever had in your life.

NOTE

- Cooking time will vary dependent on thickness of your chop. Pork chops are done when they are perfectly browned on both sides.

CHICKEN

Servings:
1
Category:
Protein
Prep time:
5 minutes
Cook time:
30-35 minutes
Total time:
40 minutes
CertifiedKetogenic.com **Rating:**
Certified Ketogenic

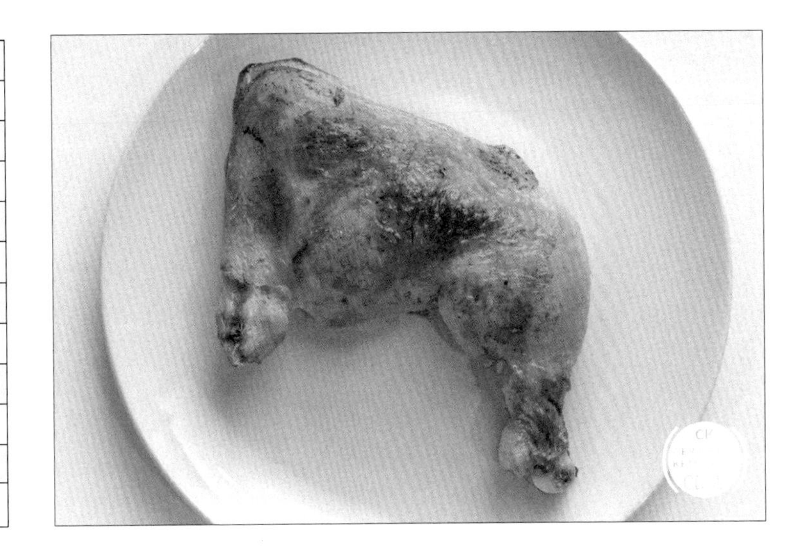

WHAT YOU NEED

1 skin-on chicken thigh

2 TBSP avocado oil

WHAT YOU DO

1. If you know how to grill a chicken leg well, go right ahead. If you're not a confident griller and / or you don't have a grill, here's how to cook a chicken thigh in your oven.
2. Preheat oven to 375°F.
3. Rinse the chicken and pat dry with kitchen towel (paper).
4. Rub avocado oil all over the chicken and place skin side down in an oiled roasting pan.
5. Roast for 20 to 25 minutes.
6. Carefully flip the chicken so that the skin is on the top and roast 10 more minutes.

BUNLESS BURGERS

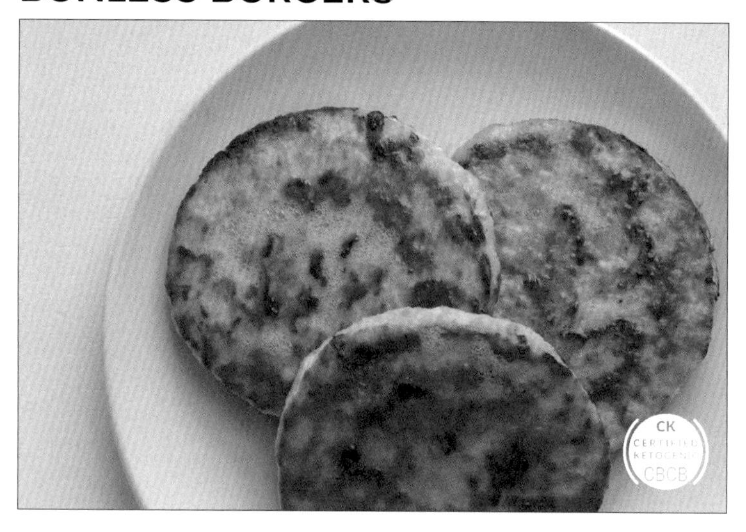

Servings:
1
Category:
Protein
Prep time:
0 minutes
Cook time:
10 minutes
Total time:
10 minutes
CertifiedKetogenic.com **Rating:**
Certified Ketogenic

WHAT YOU NEED

¼ lb / 4 oz burger, whichever meat you prefer

WHAT YOU DO

1. Grill or pan-fry your burger per the instructions on the manufacturer's packaging.

NOTES

- Burgers aren't just for Summer anymore! This recipe is so easy and versatile, you'll no doubt incorporate it into your keto lifestyle long after the 28-Day Challenge is over.
- When pan-frying your burger, you can grease the pan with reserved bacon fat for extra flavor.
- Pick the burger meat you prefer: beef, turkey, salmon... your meat department might have other options to choose from, too! Just avoid added ingredients.
- Whenever you have a choice, go for the higher fat percentages (for example, 75/25 beef). You'll save money, and get all that fantastic flavor! If you know a butcher, you can even ask them to grind you a fattier mincemeat.
- Costco make an excellent turkey burger that has only meat, salt and pepper and herbs in. If you are not near a Costco, look for a similar turkey burger in your local stores.
- Costco also have an excellent Salmon Burger containing nothing but salmon and seasonings.

SIDES

Prepare your taste buds for some of the most delicious sides you've ever had! These recipes are bursting with flavor. We wouldn't blame you if you just wanted to eat these for dinner (provided you've gotten in some quality protein at another meal).

ORANGE PECAN BRUSSELS & CABBAGE

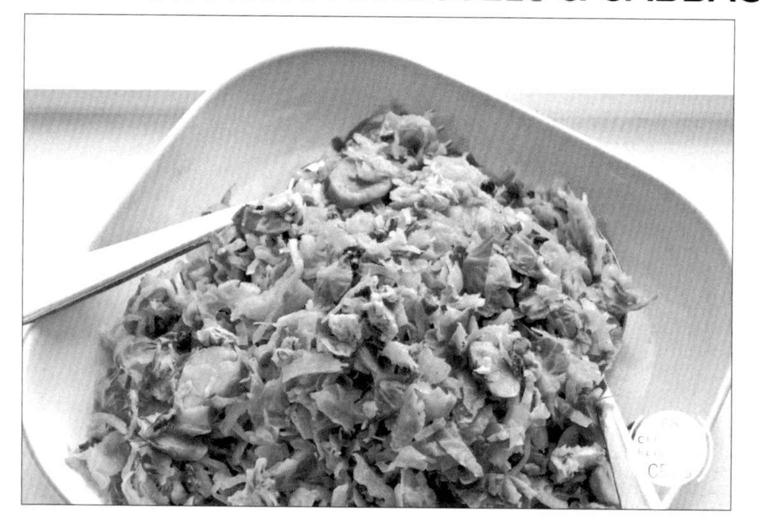

Servings:
2
Category:
Sides
Prep time:
5 minutes
Cook time:
15 minutes
Total time:
20 minutes
CertifiedKetogenic.com **Rating:**
Certified Ketogenic

WHAT YOU NEED

4 oz / 110 g butter, softened

zest of ½ orange

juice of ½ orange

½ tsp orange extract

½ tsp sea salt

ground black pepper

1 oz / 30 g pecans, toasted and finely chopped

2 ½ oz / 70 g Brussels Sprouts, shredded

2 ½ oz / 70 g cabbage, shredded

¼ cup / 2 fl oz water

WHAT YOU DO

1. In a bowl, mix together the butter, orange zest and juice, orange extract, sea salt, pepper and pecans until completely combined. It takes a little effort to bring it all together. Hang in there.
2. Place the Brussels, cabbage and water in a large pan over medium-high heat and cook for about 12 - 15 minutes, until crisp-tender. You do not want soggy greens.
3. Drain vegetables really well and return to the hot pan. Add ¼ of the orange pecan butter and toss the greens well until completely coated

NOTES

- This recipe makes enough butter mix for three additional batches. Put the extra into a plastic freezer bag and shape it into a little parcel before freezing, or roll in cling wrap and freeze in an airtight container.
- This butter mix also tastes great served on roasted chicken! Butter is the best!

HOT BACON & CABBAGE SLAW

Servings:
2
Category:
Sides
Prep time:
5 minutes
Cook time:
12 minutes
Total time:
17 minutes
CertifiedKetogenic.com **Rating:**
Certified Ketogenic

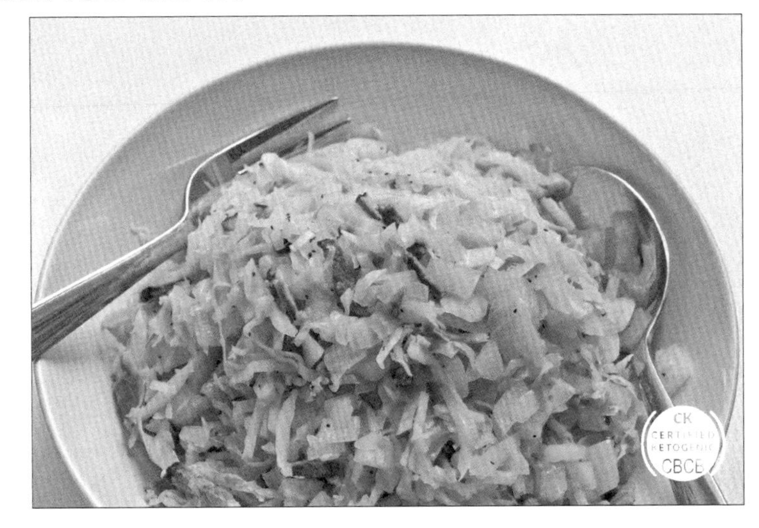

WHAT YOU NEED

1 slice (rasher) bacon, finely chopped

2 ½ oz / 70 g onion, finely chopped

5 oz / 140 g cabbage, shredded

1 ½ tsp apple cider vinegar (we use Bragg's)

⅛ tsp celery seed

⅛ tsp sea salt

½ oz / 15 g xylitol

WHAT YOU DO

1. In a large pan, sauté the bacon and onion over a medium heat for about 5 minutes until the bacon is lightly browned and the onion is just starting to soften.
2. Add the cabbage to the pan, stir well, and cook, stirring frequently, for about 5 minutes until the cabbage is crisp-tender.
3. Add the vinegar, celery seed, sea salt, and xylitol, and stirring well, cook for 1 minute.

SMOKY CREAMED MUSHROOMS

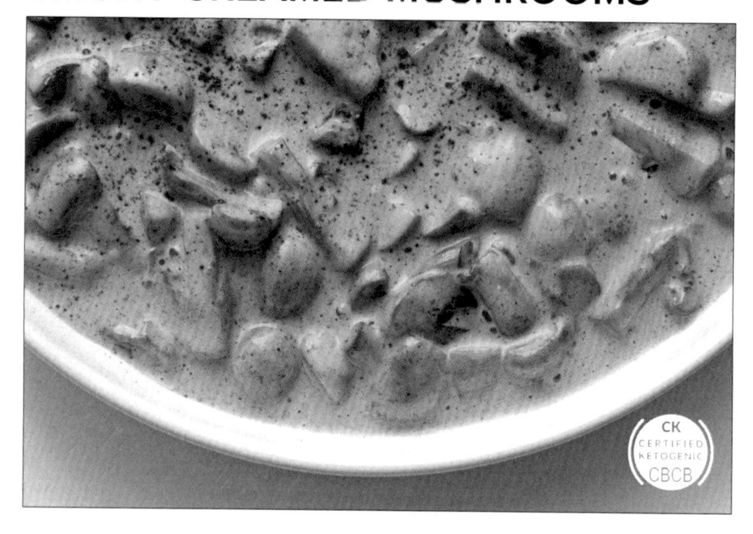

Servings:
2
Category:
Sides
Prep time:
5 minutes
Cook time:
5 minutes
Total time:
10 minutes
CertifiedKetogenic.com **Rating:**
Certified Ketogenic

WHAT YOU NEED

¾ oz / 20 g butter

6 oz / 170 g button mushrooms, quartered

¼ tsp konjac flour

¼ cup / 2 fl oz chicken stock

¼ cup / 2 fl oz heavy cream

¾ tsp smoked paprika

¼ tsp sea salt

WHAT YOU DO

1. Melt the butter in a skillet, add the mushrooms and sauté for 3 minutes – until just cooked on the cut edges.
2. Remove the mushrooms from the pan and reserve.
3. In a small bowl place the konjac flour, and whisking continuously, pour in the stock and then the heavy cream until completely combined.
4. Pour the stock mixture into the skillet, and stirring constantly, heat until thickened.
5. Add the smoked paprika, sea salt, and reserved mushrooms to the skillet and stir well. Cook for 1 minute to heat the mushrooms through. Try not to eat them before you get them to the table.

LEEK & CAULIFLOWER RISOTTO

Servings:
2
Category:
Sides
Prep time:
5 minutes
Cook time:
15 minutes
Total time:
20 minutes
CertifiedKetogenic.com **Rating:**
Certified Ketogenic

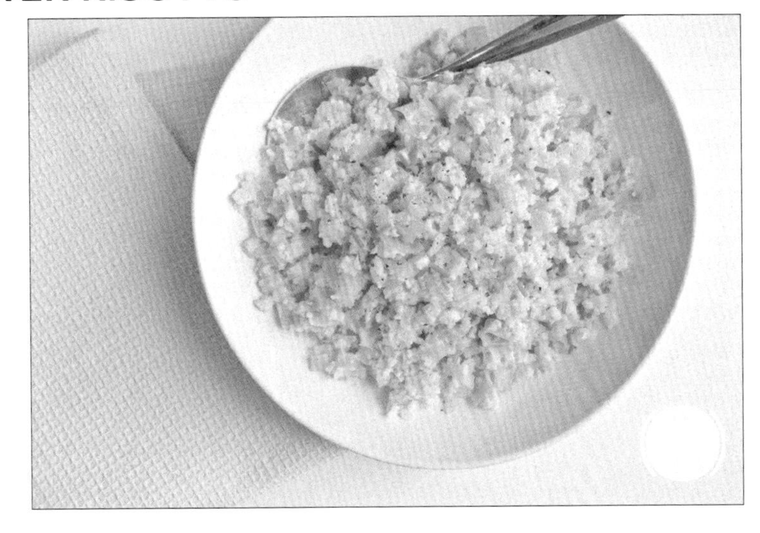

WHAT YOU NEED

1 TBSP avocado oil

8 oz / 225 g leeks, finely sliced

½ cup / 4 fl oz chicken stock

sea salt

ground black pepper

8 oz / 225 g riced cauliflower

handful of chives for garnish, chopped

WHAT YOU DO

1. Melt the avocado oil in a large skillet over high heat. Add the finely sliced leeks and reduce the heat to medium. Sauté the leeks until they are soft, about 10 minutes.
2. Add the stock, sea salt, and pepper, and stir well.
3. Once the stock starts to simmer, add the riced cauliflower and stir well.
4. Cook for 3 to 5 minutes until the cauliflower is just tender, stirring occasionally. Do not overcook as the cauliflower will turn to mush. We're not trying to make mash here.
5. Remove from the heat, stir well and spoon into a serving dish.
6. Garnish with fresh chives.

LEMON HAZELNUT LEEKS

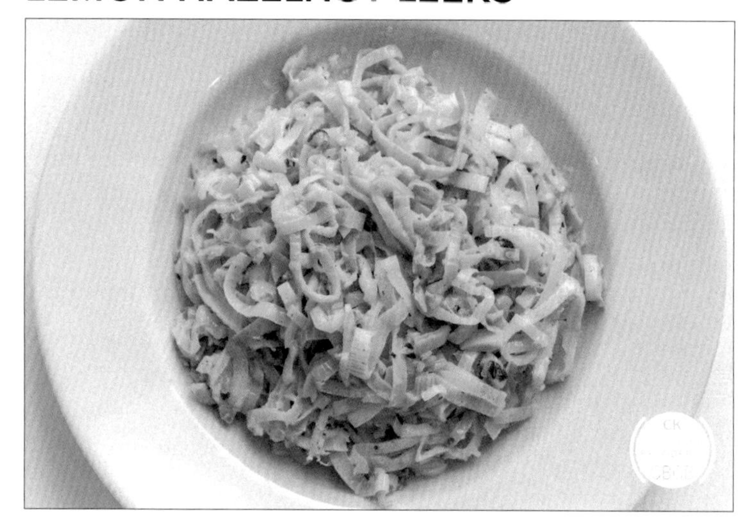

Servings:
2
Category:
Sides
Prep time:
5 minutes
Cook time:
10 minutes
Total time:
15 minutes
CertifiedKetogenic.com **Rating:**
Certified Ketogenic

WHAT YOU NEED

4 oz / 110 g butter, softened

zest of ½ lemon

juice of ½ lemon

¼ tsp sea salt

ground black pepper

2 ¾ oz / 75 g hazelnuts, toasted and finely chopped

1 TBSP avocado oil

8 oz / 225 g leeks, trimmed and finely sliced

WHAT YOU DO

1. In a bowl, mix together the butter, lemon zest and juice, sea salt, pepper and hazelnuts until completely combined.
2. Heat the avocado oil in a pan and sauté the finely sliced leeks over medium-low heat for about 8 minutes until soft.
3. Add ¼ of the Lemon Hazelnut Butter to the pan and toss the leeks until the butter has melted and completely mixed in.

NOTES

- This recipe makes enough butter mix for three additional batches. Put the extra into a plastic freezer bag and shape it into a little parcel before freezing, or roll in cling wrap and freeze in an airtight container.
- This butter mix also tastes great served on roasted or grilled meat! Butter is the best!

CELERY & CUCUMBER SALAD WITH HERBS

Servings:
2
Category:
Sides
Prep time:
15 minutes
Cook time:
0 minutes
Total time:
15 minutes
CertifiedKetogenic.com **Rating:**
Certified Ketogenic

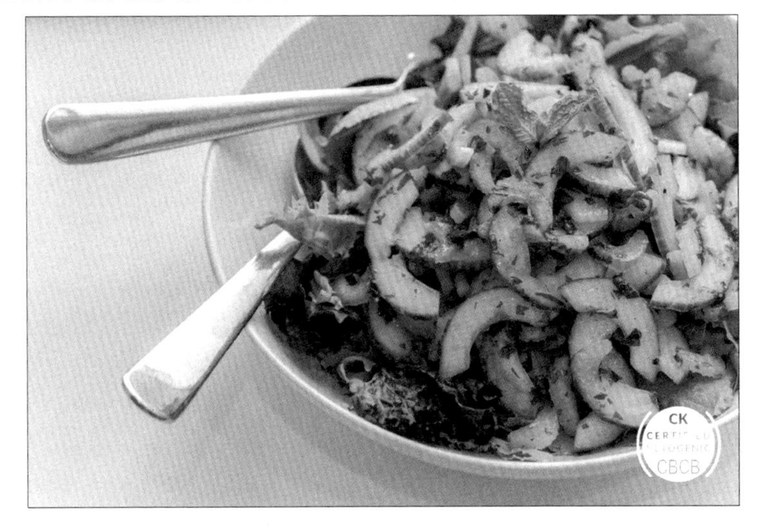

WHAT YOU NEED

¼ large English cucumber

1 celery stalk, thinly sliced crosswise

⅛ oz / 4 g coarsely chopped fresh flat-leaf parsley

⅛ oz / 4 g coarsely chopped fresh mint

1 TBSP avocado oil

½ bag of mixed salad greens

coarse sea salt

freshly ground black pepper

WHAT YOU DO

1. Peel the cucumber with a peeler. Cut off the ends. Cut the whole cucumber in half crosswise. Cut each piece in half lengthwise. Run a teaspoon down the center of the cucumber to cleanly and easily remove the seeds, leaving you with hollowed out cucumber "boats". Then slice thinly crosswise.
2. Toss the sliced celery, sliced cucumber, chopped parsley and mint, plus the avocado oil into a bowl and mix thoroughly.
3. In a shallow serving dish or platter spread a bed of the mixed salad greens.
4. Spoon the celery / cucumber mixture over the greens leaving the salad around the edge of the dish uncovered.
5. Season with salt and pepper and garnish with sprigs of parsley and mint.

AVOCADO & WALNUT SALAD

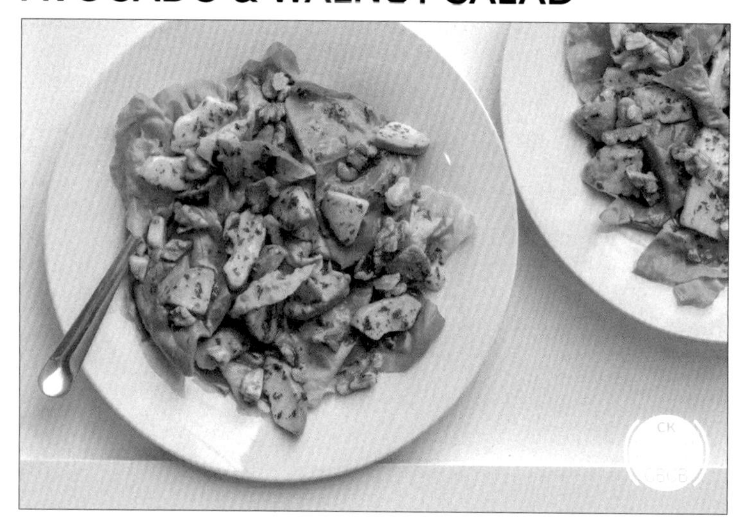

Servings:
2
Category:
Sides
Prep time:
10 minutes
Cook time:
0 minutes
Total time:
10 minutes
CertifiedKetogenic.com **Rating:**
Certified Ketogenic

WHAT YOU NEED

1 Butter or Bibb lettuce

4 TBSP extra virgin olive oil

1 ½ TBSP xylitol

2 TBSP white wine vinegar

1 TBSP finely chopped fresh parsley

¼ tsp dried oregano

coarse sea salt and ground pepper

1 avocado

2 oz / 55 g shelled walnuts, chopped into large pieces

WHAT YOU DO

1. Tear the lettuce into large pieces and place in a serving dish or bowl.
2. Whisk the olive oil, xylitol, white wine vinegar, parsley, and oregano in a small bowl until completely blended and the xylitol dissolved. Season with salt and pepper to taste.
3. Cut the avocados in half lengthwise, remove the stone, peel, and then slice neatly into pieces.
4. Add avocado pieces to the dressing and carefully turn to coat them completely. Spoon the avocado slices evenly over the bed of lettuce. Drizzle the remaining dressing over the salad and then sprinkle the walnuts evenly on top.

BACON PARMESAN BRUSSELS SPROUTS

Servings:
2
Category:
Sides
Prep time:
5 minutes
Cook time:
10 minutes
Total time:
15 minutes
CertifiedKetogenic.com **Rating:**
Certified Ketogenic

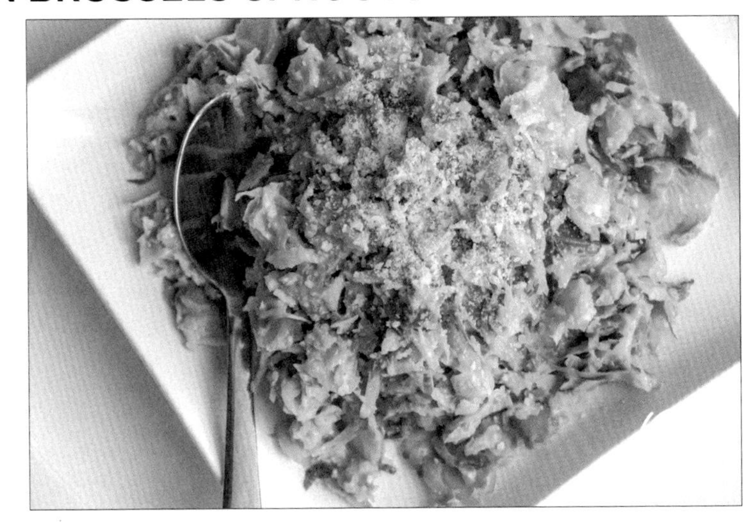

WHAT YOU NEED

2 oz / 55 g bacon

4 oz / 110 g butter, softened

½ oz / 15 g Parmesan, finely grated

½ tsp onion powder

5 oz / 140 g Brussels Sprouts, shredded

¼ cup / 2 fl oz water

WHAT YOU DO

1. Cook the bacon to your preferred crispiness. Chop or crumble.
2. In a bowl, mix together the butter, bacon, Parmesan and onion powder until completely combined. It takes a little effort to bring it all together. Hang in there.
3. Place the Brussels and water in a pan over medium-high heat and cook for about 10 minutes, until crisp-tender. You do not want soggy Brussels.
4. Drain Brussels really well and return to the hot pan. Add ¼ of the bacon Parmesan butter and toss the Brussels well until completely coated.

NOTES

- This recipe makes enough butter mix for three additional batches. Put the extra into a plastic freezer bag and shape it into a little parcel before freezing, or roll in cling wrap and freeze in an airtight container.
- This butter mix also tastes great served on roasted or grilled meat! Butter is the best!

CILANTRO LIME BROCCOLI

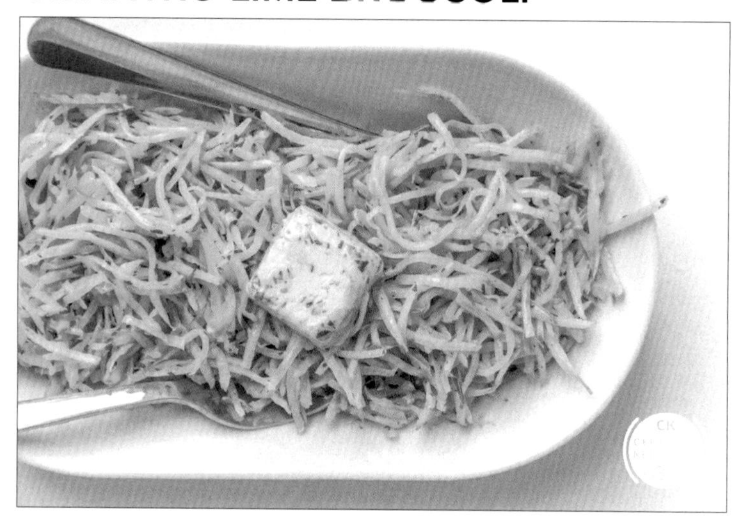

Servings:
2
Category:
Sides
Prep time:
5 minutes
Cook time:
8 minutes
Total time:
13 minutes
CertifiedKetogenic.com **Rating:**
Certified Ketogenic

WHAT YOU NEED

4 oz / 110 g butter, softened

zest of 1 lime

1 TBSP lime juice

⅛ tsp sea salt

1 ½ TBSP fresh cilantro, finely chopped

1 TBSP avocado oil

5 oz / 140 g broccoli slaw (pre-bagged in store)

WHAT YOU DO

1. In a bowl, mix together the butter, lime zest and juice, sea salt, and fresh cilantro until completely combined.
2. Heat the avocado oil in a pan and sauté the broccoli slaw over medium heat for about 8 minutes until just softened.
3. Add ¼ of the Lime Cilantro Butter to the pan and toss the broccoli slaw until the butter has melted and is completely mixed in.

NOTES

- This recipe makes enough butter mix for three additional batches. Put the extra into a plastic freezer bag and shape it into a little parcel before freezing, or roll in cling wrap and freeze in an airtight container.
- This butter mix also tastes great served on roasted or grilled meat! Butter is the best!

AVOCADO LIME ZOODLES

Servings:
2
Category:
Sides
Prep time:
0 minutes
Cook time:
10 minutes
Total time:
10 minutes
CertifiedKetogenic.com **Rating:**
Certified Ketogenic

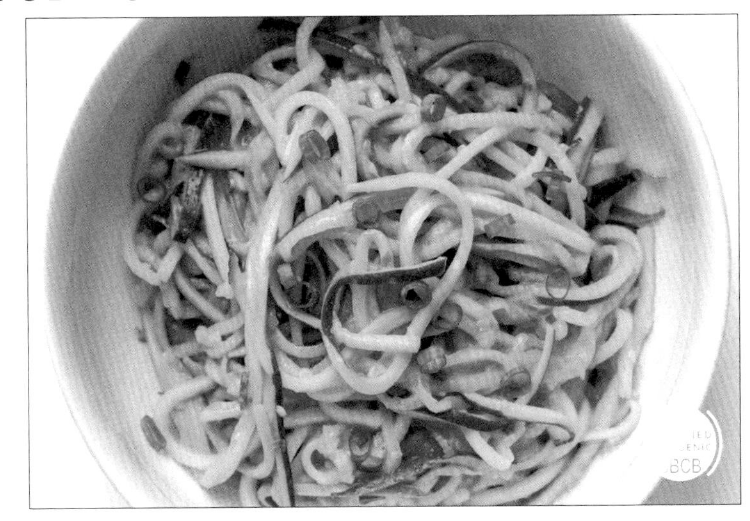

WHAT YOU NEED

½ avocado

¾ tsp lime juice

4 oz / 110 g butter, softened

½ scallion (green or spring onion), very finely sliced

⅛ tsp sea salt

6 oz / 170 g zucchini

1 TBSP avocado oil

WHAT YOU DO

1. Cut the avocado in half lengthwise, remove the stone, peel, chop roughly into pieces and then toss in a bowl with the lime juice until all pieces are completely coated.
2. In a bowl, mash together the butter and avocado lime mixture until completely combined.
3. Stir in the finely chopped onion and the sea salt and mix until blended evenly.
4. Make zoodles from the zucchini by using a spiralizer or a simple julienne peeler. If you have neither, just sliced the zucchini very finely into thin sticks.
5. Heat the avocado oil in a pan and sauté the zucchini over medium heat for about 3 to 4 minutes until barely soft.
6. Add ¼ of the avocado lime butter to the pan and toss the zoodles gently until the butter has melted and is completely mixed in.

NOTES

- This recipe makes enough butter mix for three additional batches. Put the extra into a plastic freezer bag and shape it into a little parcel before freezing, or roll in cling wrap and freeze in an airtight container.
- This butter mix also tastes great served on roasted or grilled meat! Butter is the best!

ROSEMARY OLIVE CABBAGE

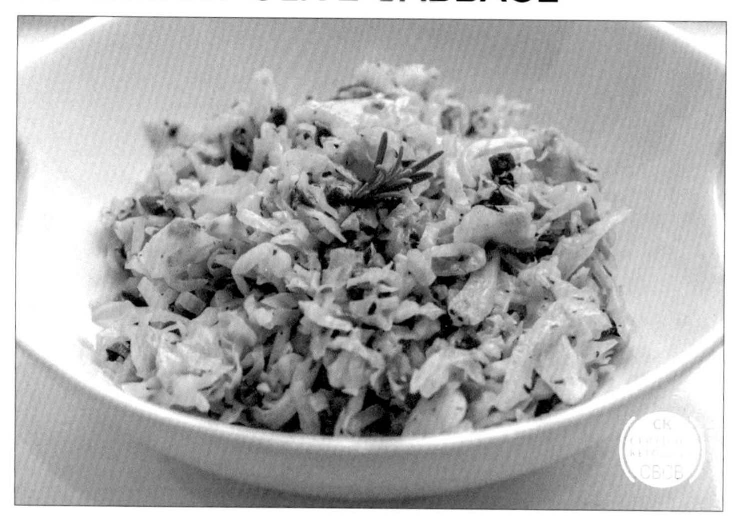

Servings:
2
Category:
Sides
Prep time:
10 minutes
Cook time:
10 minutes
Total time:
20 minutes
CertifiedKetogenic.com **Rating:**
Certified Ketogenic

WHAT YOU NEED

4 oz / 110 g butter, softened

2 oz / 55 g black olives, pitted and finely chopped

1 TBSP fresh rosemary, very finely chopped

5 oz / 140 g cabbage, shredded

¼ cup / 2 fl oz water

WHAT YOU DO

1. In a bowl, mix together the butter, chopped olives and finely chopped fresh rosemary until completely combined. It takes a little effort to bring it all together. Hang in there.
2. Stir in the finely chopped onion and the sea salt and mix until blended evenly through the butter.
3. Place the shredded cabbage and water in a pan over medium-high heat and cook for about 10 minutes, until crisp-tender. You do not want soggy cabbage.
4. Drain cabbage really well and return to the hot pan. Add ¼ of the rosemary olive butter and toss the cabbage well until completely coated.

NOTES

- This recipe makes enough butter mix for three additional batches. Put the extra into a plastic freezer bag and shape it into a little parcel before freezing, or roll in cling wrap and freeze in an airtight container.
- This butter mix also tastes great served on roasted or grilled meat! Butter is the best!

MUSHROOM RISOTTO

Servings:
2
Category:
Sides
Prep time:
0 minutes
Cook time:
10 minutes
Total time:
10 minutes
CertifiedKetogenic.com **Rating:**
Certified Ketogenic

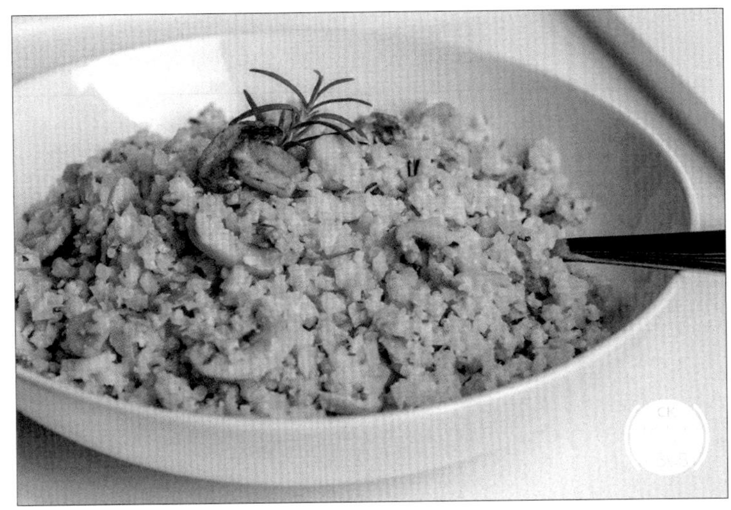

WHAT YOU NEED

1 TBSP avocado oil

5 oz / 140 g riced cauliflower

4 oz / 110 g mushrooms, sliced

1 ½ oz / 42 g Parmesan, finely grated

½ TBSP fresh rosemary, finely chopped

WHAT YOU DO

1. Melt the avocado oil in a large skillet over medium heat. Add the riced cauliflower and sliced mushrooms and sauté for about 8 - 10 minutes, stirring frequently until they are just soft.
2. Stir in the finely grated Parmesan and chopped fresh rosemary and stir gently until everything is completely combined.
3. Remove from the heat and spoon into a serving dish.

AVOCADO FETA SALAD

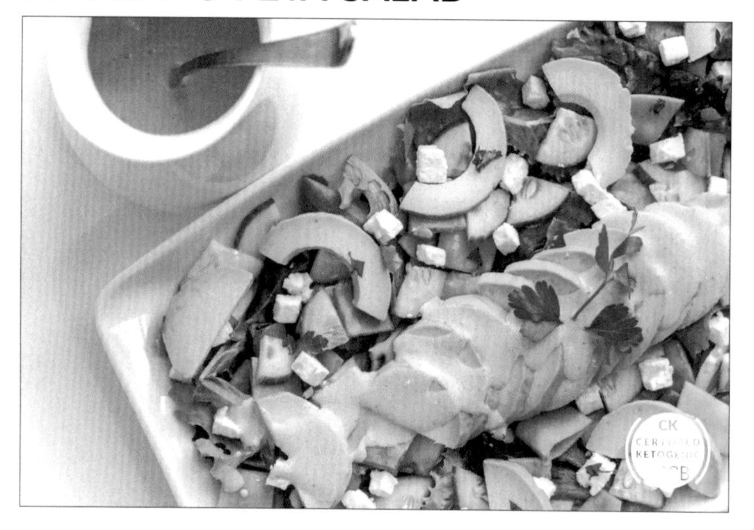

Servings:
2
Category:
Sides
Prep time:
15 minutes
Cook time:
0 minutes
Total time:
15 minutes
CertifiedKetogenic.com **Rating:**
Certified Ketogenic

WHAT YOU NEED

¼ cup / 2 fl oz plain, unsweetened full-fat Greek yogurt (Non-fat will not work!)

¼ cup / 2 fl oz sour cream

½ TBSP lime juice

½ TBSP apple cider vinegar

¼ oz / 7 g fresh parsley

2 large fresh basil leaves

2 scallions (green onions / spring onions)

⅛ tsp sea salt

⅛ tsp ground black pepper

mixed lettuce greens

¼ English cucumber, quartered and sliced

1 ¾ oz / 45 g snow peas, cut into bite-sized pieces

2 oz / 55 g feta cheese, cut into small cubes

½ avocado, halved lengthwise, stone removed, peeled, and sliced

WHAT YOU DO

1. Place yogurt and sour cream in a blender and blend well. Add lime juice, apple cider vinegar, parsley, basil, onions, sea salt and pepper to the blender and blend until completely smooth and green.
2. Toss together the mixed lettuce greens, cut snow peas, and sliced cucumber and pile onto a plate or serving dish. Sprinkle the feta cubes over the vegetables, then lay avocado slices on top.
3. Pour dressing over the salad and serve immediately. Keep leftover dressing in an airtight jar in the 'fridge.

CRUNCHY WINTER SLAW

Servings:
2
Category:
Sides
Prep time:
15 minutes
Standing time:
30 minutes
Total time:
45 minutes
CertifiedKetogenic.com **Rating:**
Certified Ketogenic

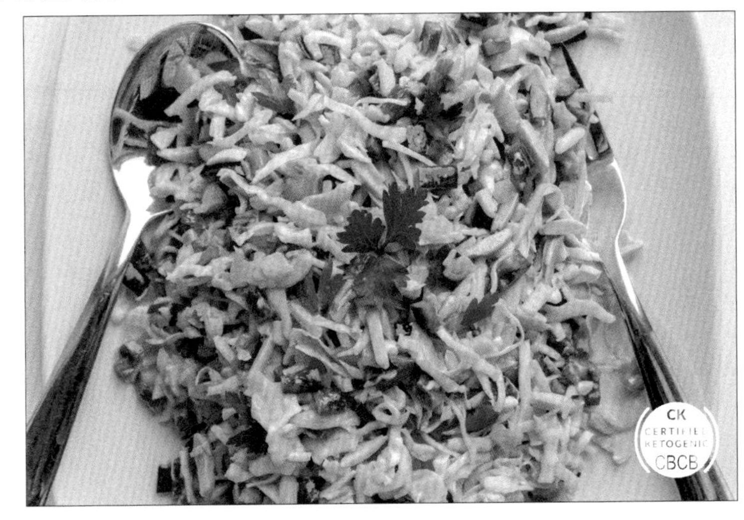

WHAT YOU NEED

3 TBSP / 1 ½ fl oz avocado oil

2 TBSP / 1 fl oz apple cider vinegar

2 tsp Dijon mustard

1 TBSP xylitol

¼ tsp sea salt

2 oz / 55 g onion, finely chopped

5 oz / 140 g cabbage, shredded

1 ½ oz / 42 g toasted slivered almonds

1 ½ oz / 42 g red pepper, sliced and cut into pieces

½ oz / 15 g fresh parsley, coarsely chopped

sea salt

ground black pepper

WHAT YOU DO

1. Place avocado oil, apple cider vinegar, mustard, xylitol, and sea salt in a bowl and whisk well. Add the finely chopped onion and leave to stand for at least 30 minutes before serving.
2. Toss the shredded cabbage, toasted silvered almonds, red pepper pieces, and coarsely chopped fresh parsley in a bowl.
3. Pour the dressing over the salad and toss well until cabbage is completely coated.

FAT BOMBS

Many keto nutrition guides, in our opinion, over-emphasize what's known as the "fat bomb" – a delightful confection which delivers comfort-food taste with a wham-pow of added fat.

There are, however, down-sides to fat bombs which are often understated.

1. They encourage dependence on the concept of "dessert," a holdover form of snacking from our SAD lifestyle better left behind.

2. They trigger some of the same reward centers of our brain so we tend to remain addicted to those sweets and treats they are designed to replace.

3. Small and delicious, they are easy to overeat if you have trouble with awareness of your body's hunger signals.

That said, if you struggle to eat keto-levels of fat, a fat bomb might be just the thing to help. Add one to Meal 3 and eat it with the meal rather than waiting in between (this is so your insulin only has to respond once to the needs of your digestion).

Please note the fat bombs are not built into the meal plans or shoppings lists.

If you find any of the warning above speaks to a personal struggle with which you are all-too-familiar, it's good to be honest with yourself and skip the fat bombs. They can help, but they're not necessary, especially if they will cause you to struggle with a known addictive personality.

LEMON CHEESECAKE FAT BOMBS

Servings:
45
Category:
Fat Bombs
Cook time:
10 minutes
Standing time:
2 hours in freezer
Total time:
10 minutes + 2-hour wait to eat
CertifiedKetogenic.com **Rating:**
Certified Ketogenic

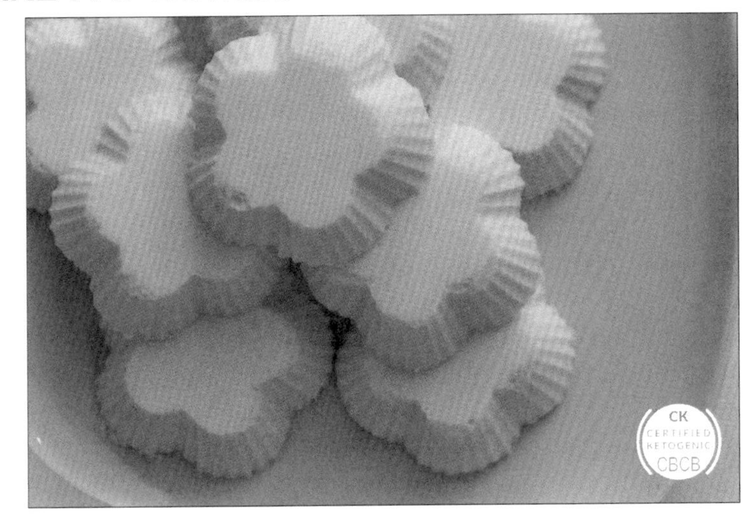

WHAT YOU NEED

4 oz / 110 g butter

4 oz / 110 g coconut oil

3 TBSP powdered xylitol (or pulverize granular xylitol in a high-speed blender)

4 oz / 110 g cream cheese

zest of 1 lemon

2-3 TBSP lemon juice (depending on how lemony you like)

WHAT YOU DO

1. Put butter and coconut oil in a pan over low heat. Sieve the powdered xylitol directly into the pan to make sure there's no lumps and stir until fat is melted and xylitol completely dissolved.
2. Add cream cheese and stir over low heat until completely melted.
3. Add lemon zest and juice and stir well.
4. Transfer to a jug and carefully pour into silicone molds supported on a cookie sheet.
5. Carefully carry the cookie sheet to the freezer and put in the freezer on a level surface.
6. Allow to freeze – at least 2 hours before enjoying. Once frozen, remove from the molds and store in an airtight container in the freezer.
7. Either eat straight from the freezer or leave to warm up for 5 minutes before eating.

NOTES

- How many pieces you get out of a batch depends on the size of your mold or ice cube tray. The smaller the molds, the better, as it's better to eat two smaller fat bombs if you need them than eat a larger one that is too much.

CHOCOLATE BUTTER CUPS

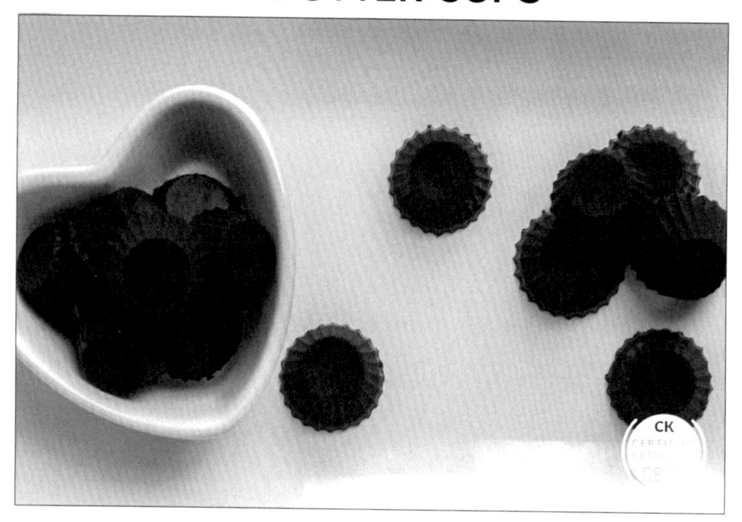

Servings:
30
Category:
Fat Bombs
Cook time:
10 minutes
Standing time:
2 hours in freezer
Total time:
10 minutes + 2-hour wait to eat
CertifiedKetogenic.com **Rating:**
Certified Ketogenic

WHAT YOU NEED

8 oz / 225 g butter OR ghee

1 ½ oz powdered xylitol (or pulverize granular xylitol in a high-speed blender)

½ oz cocoa powder

2 oz / 30 g 100% unsweetened chocolate, finely chopped

WHAT YOU DO

1. Put the butter or ghee in a small pan over a low heat. Sieve the powdered xylitol and then the cocoa powder directly into the pan to make sure there's no lumps, and then stir until the butter is melted and xylitol and cocoa powder are completely dissolved.
2. Add the chopped chocolate and stir until chocolate is completely melted and mixed in.
3. Transfer to a jug and carefully pour into silicone molds supported on a cookie sheet.
4. Carefully carry the cookie sheet to the freezer and put in the freezer on a level surface.
5. Allow to freeze – at least 2 hours before enjoying. Once frozen, remove from the molds and store in an airtight container in the freezer.
6. Either eat straight from the freezer or leave to warm up for a minute before eating. These melt very easily.

NOTES

- How many pieces you get out of a batch depends on the size of your mold or ice cube tray. The smaller the molds, the better, as it's better to eat two smaller fat bombs if you need them than eat a larger one that is too much.

PART 5: LONG-TERM HEALTH

Congratulations on completing this 28-day course! Way to kickass!

We know this was a dramatic shift in your lifestyle, and at times it may have seemed easier to quit.

If you've reached this point, implementing the tenets of this book and following the nutrition plan without deviation,
Day 29 no doubt finds you feeling the amazing effects of having switched on the fat-burning mechanisms of your body.

But now we're at the end of the book, and you may be wondering where you take your keto journey from here. The changes you've made to your lifestyle and diet should not be limited to this 28-day program. This program is designed to kick-start a lifestyle change which will help you reach even bigger weight loss and wellness goals.

Keto is safe and effective for the long term. You already know where your old lifestyle got you, so keep it keto and keep feeling the benefits!

Read on for some tips and guidelines, and have no fear.

DAY 29 & BEYOND

The important thing now is to keep going! Your body will flourish if you continue to follow the keto guidelines you've learned during the past four weeks.

One option you have, if you are the type who likes to have a guide to follow in everything, is to return to the start of this book and repeat everything for another 28 days, as many times as you like. If you've identified favorite portions of this book, and you don't require a lot of variety, you can build your own weekly menu and fitness plan and just stick to that until you feel ready to change it up.

If you feel adventurous and are ready to venture into the wider world of ketogenic living, there's a lot of information out there. In the following chapter, you'll find links to online resources from our team of keto experts, including Facebook groups to provide community, podcasts to provide the latest information and encouragement, recipes for new things to try throughout the year, and resources to help you navigate the rest of your life from a ketogenic approach.

We recommend you keep tracking until all this keto "stuff" feels natural and you know the tricks and methods which help you feel your best. But, even if you find you no longer need to track your food consumption, we hope you'll see the value of, and never stop, practicing regular self-evaluation, mindfulness, and revisiting your goals to assess your progress. Return to this book every now and then to shore up your foundations if you experience overwhelm.

ADJUSTING PRIORITIES

For almost a month, you've made the right choice to prioritize a healthy lifestyle. Keeping up this shift in mindset will help you continue to build on the progress you've already made. Continue to prioritize nutrition and exercise going forward.

A rolling stone gathers no moss. We are creatures of habit, and that's why all the work to build healthy habits sets you up for success. On the other hand, if you get into a routine without keeping your goals in mind, forward momentum can come to a stop. Make your number one goal self-awareness. Whenever you recognize something you're doing isn't building a better, stronger you, take the time to re-evaluate, and adjust. Incorporate the habits you've built as you go forward, building yourself up, rather than stripping everything away and starting from scratch over and over again.

Become a scientist who researches your own health. Try new things and see how they make you feel. Always be limber, agile, ready to shift approaches and figure out what works best for you.

Spoiler: it may not be what everyone else is doing.

TIPS FOR SUCCESS

Asking you to do something "by the book" for 28 days is one thing, but setting you free to go about the rest of your life means you're going to encounter situations which aren't ideal, no matter how prepared you think you are.

Here are our tips to keep up the good habits you've developed and keep you on track toward your long-term goals.

Eating Out

Now that you have completed your Kickass Keto challenge, you may be interested in eating out socially again, but are concerned about what choices to make from the restaurant menu. We understand! Nothing seems to stress out our Facebook members more than the thought of ordering food at a restaurant where the preparation is out of their control.

But there are some simple things which can help. Print out the Keto-Friendly Ingredients List from this book, or keep your digital copy of this book on your mobile device, so you can access it anywhere. Keeping this resource handy will help you if things start to get confusing.

The key, when eating out, is to avoid starches, wheats, and sugars. Any prepared sauce is suspect until you've seen an ingredient list. Never be afraid to ask to speak directly to the chef if you have questions, and remember a protein and a simple steamed vegetable with butter are usually a safe bet.

Many keto people find the most reliable options when eating out are a bunless bacon cheeseburger (with a real cheese like Cheddar or Swiss, not American cheese product), or a steak. Most restaurants offer some kind of steamed veggies to which you can add butter, and substitutions are often free or only a small up-charge.

The nice thing about keto is if we skip a meal, our blood sugar won't send us on a mine cart ride with a crash at the end. You can always simply order a water, tea, or coffee, and enjoy the company you're with, and eat when you get home. Your health is at stake, and eating something of dubious quality isn't worth it.

Keto doesn't need to be confusing, or overwhelming. Keto is, really, about as simple as it gets. Once you understand the science of why keto helps, knowing what food to choose becomes easier.

And just because you're at the end of the book doesn't mean we at Ketovangelist don't have more help to offer you. Our podcasts, blog posts, and Facebook groups are full of information to help you fully immerse yourself in a keto way of life.

A Note About Expectations

One thing to note is that a keto newcomer will often experience a very abrupt and dramatic weight loss after switching from a SAD lifestyle. This is a result of inflammation and water retention which quickly dispel when insulin and blood sugar levels are kept under control. You may not have noticed, but the delicious meal plan also eliminated a lot of unhealthy processed ingredients such as grains and vegetable oils, and this only increased the inflammation-reductive effects.

Once you have eliminated the majority of inflammation and retained water, your weight loss will slow. You may even reach what is colloquially known as a "stall" among dieters. These are normal processes, and do not indicate you are doing anything wrong.

Your body will use the newfound nutrition and energy to heal a lot of systems in your body. It starts with inflammation because of how damaging it is, and the weight loss is a delightful byproduct. Next, your body may focus on joint pain, or nervous system repair, your immune system, or hormone balances. These things are difficult to track, especially if you only follow a scale.

Be aware of the different ways in which your life will improve: mood, pain, energy, resistance to pesky colds and viruses, improved sleep, focus, and outlook. Make notes about these other less common metrics as you continue to track your eating, habits, and exercise. Avoid the temptation to return to a normal SAD diet or incorporate cheats if you feel frustrated with the measurements on the scale or a slower drop in pant size.

You don’t have to do this alone.

The online support communities of fellow Ketovangelists will help you feel less alone, and are great resources if you find yourself feeling lost. The next page lists all of the Ketovangelist network sites, resources, podcasts, and groups so you have a circle of information that will match up with the solid foundation you've spent the last four weeks setting up.

For more dedicated advice and assistance on your keto journey, consider reaching out for help from a Ketovangelist lifestyle and nutrition coach. A coach can give you specific input about your keto lifestyle, tailored to your specific goals. You don't **need** a coach if you are on track with your goals, but if you are struggling, it's awesome to have one of our many experienced Ketovangelist Coaches in your corner.

KETOVANGELIST NETWORK RESOURCES

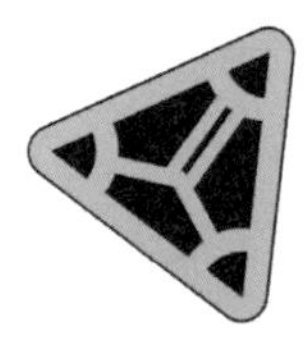

Ketovangelist – Science and Stories of Keto

Podcast: ketovangelist.com/category/podcast

Ketogenic Success Facebook Group: facebook.com/groups/ketogenicsuccess

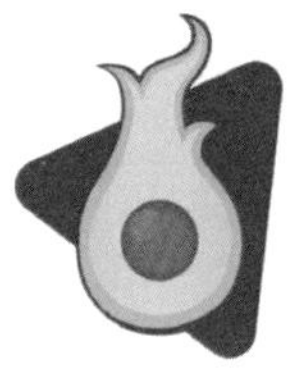

Ketovangelist Kitchen – Ketogenic Cooking

Recipes: www.ketovangelistkitchen.com

Podcast: ketovangelistkitchen.com/category/podcast

Ketovangelist Kitchen Facebook Group:
facebook.com/groups/ketovangelistkitchen

Ingredient guide: ketovangelistkitchen.com/ingredients-guide/

Cookbooks: ketovangelistkitchen.com/cookbooks-ketovangelist-kitchen

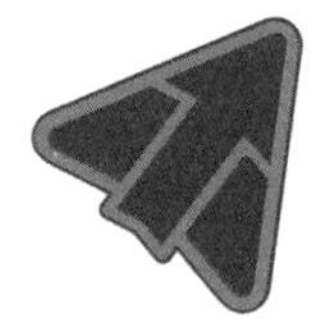

The Ketogenic Athlete – Fitness and Endurance

Podcast: theketogenicathlete.com/category/podcast

TKA Facebook Group: facebook.com/groups/theketogenicathlete

LEVELING UP YOUR KETO LIFESTYLE

Ketovangelist Unlimited
ketovangelistunlimited.com

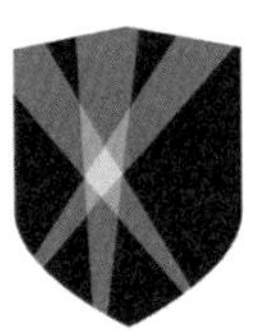

KetoCon
ketocon.org

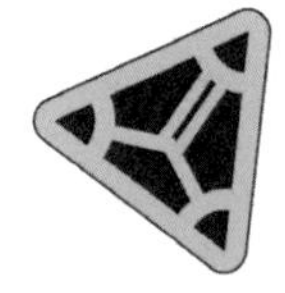

Ketovangelist Coaching
ketovangelistcoaching.com

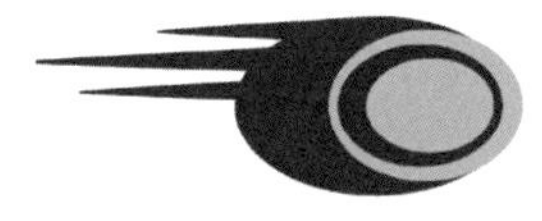

Ballistic Keto
ballisticketo.com

Certified Ketogenic
certifiedketogenic.com

ABOUT THE AUTHORS

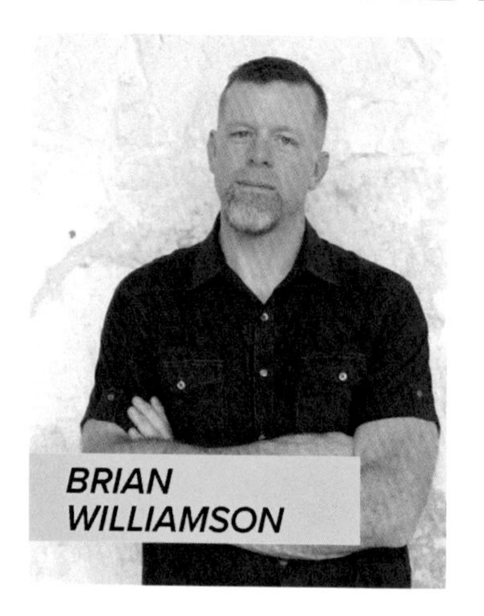

Brian is a devoted husband and father of three who discovered the ketogenic diet when researching treatments for his son's epilepsy. He learned the science behind the ketogenic way of life, and gained the tools needed to accomplish the health and fitness goals he wanted to achieve.

By adopting the ketogenic way of life, he has lost 60 pounds (so far), improved his mental and physical health, and started enjoying life.

Find Brian online at:
@ketovangelist ketovangelist.com

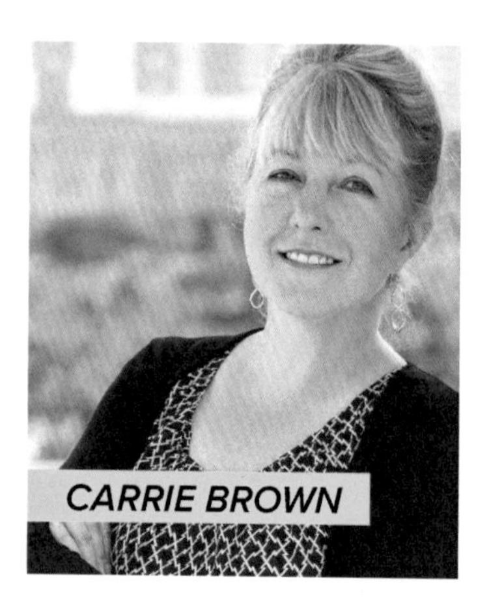

Carrie brings joy to the keto world through her wisdom, her compassion, and, of course, her incredibly delicious foods. She can often be found in the kitchen, surrounded by her four-legged friends, concocting, devising, developing, and making the impossible very possible (and affordable). When she's not there, or recording podcasts, she's excitedly zooming around the country to photograph beautiful landscapes and other living things.

Find Carrie online at:
@carrieontrippin / @lifeinthesanelane
ketovangelistkitchen.com fb.me/FlamingAvocado

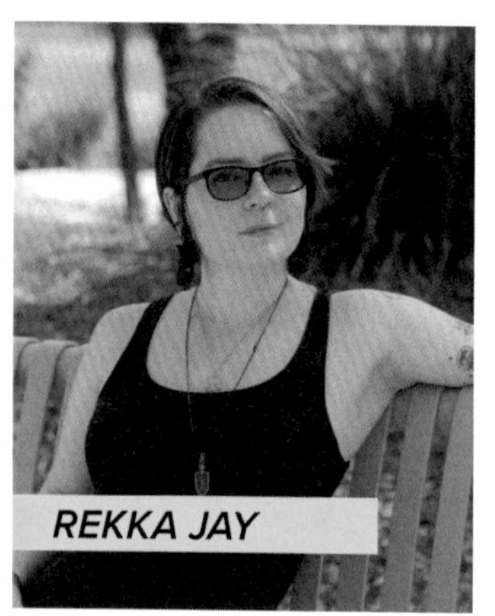

Rekka likes to keep busy, and loves how keto fuels her brain and body so she can keep going non-stop.

She's a graphic designer (both in her day job and freelance), an illustrator, fiction author, and podcast co-host. In what spare time she leaves herself, she likes to play video games, read, and then pass out on the couch with her cats.

Find Rekka online at:
Twitter & Instagram: @bittybittyzap
ketovangelist.com/author/glossbones
rjtheodore.com

Made in the USA
Middletown, DE
03 February 2018